Questions and Answers About Canine Cuisine

By Doug Bittinger
and Sandra Manes DVM
Illustrations by Donna Gregg

Published and copyrighted: Nov. 14, 2021

This book is dedicated to the memory of
Cochise: the Amazing Talking Dog
he was our first foster dog,
an invaluable mentor, and
our "Bestest Boy".

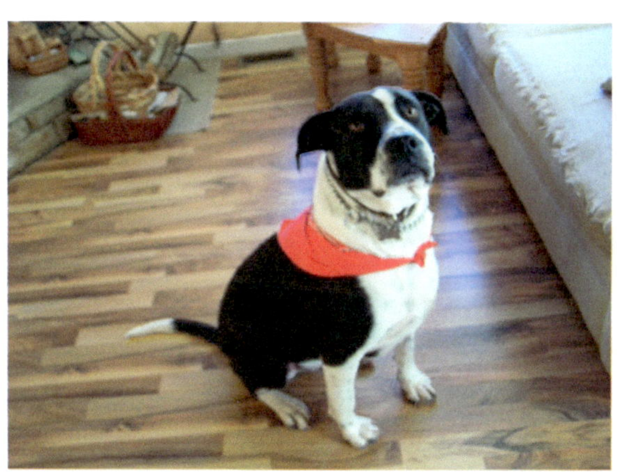

Table of Contents

About the Authors

Douglas Allan Bittinger has been an author of instructional books and magazine articles since the early 1980's. His list of publications is long. Many of his magazine articles were published under the pseudonym of Allan Douglas.

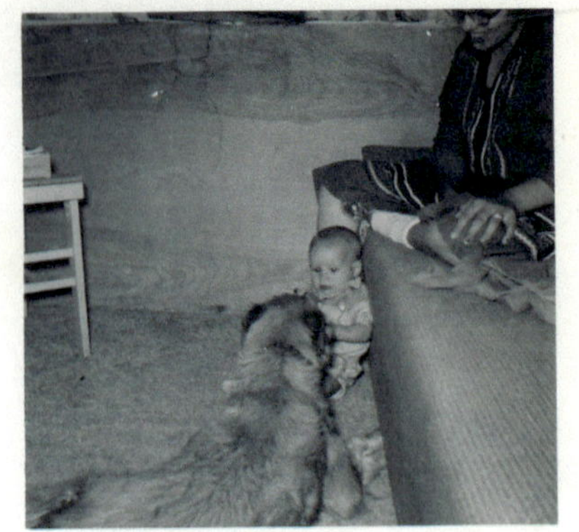

Doug has been around dogs all his life. As an infant his baby sitter and guardian was a mixed breed dog named Judy who never let him out of her sight. In 2012 Doug and his wife Marie began fostering heart worm positive dogs as they went through treatment. In 2019 that beginning became a 501(c)(3) non-profit charity dedicated to saving the lives of dogs in shelters and making them adoptable through medical and behavioral rehabilitation.

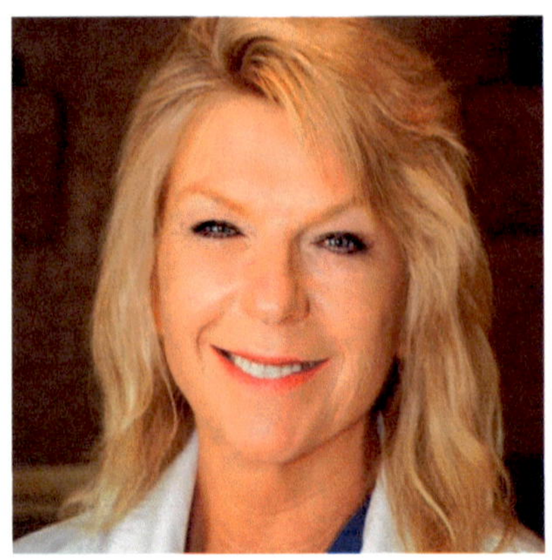

DR. SANDRA MANES D.V.M.

Education: University of Tennessee

Hometown: Newport Tennessee

Dr. Sandra Manes is a graduate of the University of Tennessee College of Veterinary Medicine. She graduated in 1996 and received the honor of graduating Magna Cum Laude. She also received her Bachelor's Degree in Animal Science from the University of Tennessee, where she graduated Summa Cum Laude in her class. She lives a very active lifestyle in which she enjoys working on her farm nestled in the foothills of East Tennessee. Her special areas of interest include avian & exotic medicine and animal behavior. In her free time she enjoys spending time with her new husband, and trying new adventurous things.

Forward

By Dr. Sandra Manes D.V.M.

If you lived through any of the commercial dog and cat food recalls, you have reason to be concerned with what you offer your pet to eat. Pet food recalls began in the later part of 1999 and have recurred again and again with excessive amounts of harmful nutrients, bacteria, chemicals and drugs which should have never reached the pet food table. The latest debate relates to Dilated Cardiomyopathy in canines and the relationship between this medical condition and feeding a gourmet or boutique diet. “We thought we were feeding the best food possible”; I have heard this comment more than once.

Doug and I have spent multiple occasions discussing pet foods. We are in agreement that we should know the source of both our human food and what we are offering our pets. Early on in a discussion with Doug about pet food, I said, if I had the time and resources I would make a wholesome food for our pets that I knew the source of products and felt comfortable feeding to my own babies and my client’s babies. Doug took those words to heart. And, here we have his well thought out, well versed, well researched book of homemade diets for dogs. Thank you, Doug Bittinger for this great source of information.

Disclaimer: No homemade diet may meet all the requirements of all life stages of the dog. It is always recommended to consult a veterinarian or veterinary nutritionist before implementing changes in a canine’s diet.

Acknowledgments

I need to recognize and thank the following for their help and guidance as I researched and wrote this book:

- Dr. Sandra Manes D.V.M.
- DogFoodAdvisor.com
- Whole Dog Journal
- Christine Filardi; certified Holistic Canine Chef
- Donna Gregg for the delightful cover and chapter illustrations see more of her work at Paint-PencilByDonna.com
- and my wife: Marie, for putting up with the mess I frequently made in her kitchen.

Introduction

As a dog person (I am reluctant to say “dog owner” because I consider dogs to be neither personal property nor livestock) I have a genuine concern for the health and well-being of my dogs. I see that they get proper medical care, and that they are sheltered, cared for, and loved.

For years we have fed the dogs a high quality kibble because it rated well with places like DogFoodAdvisor.com as far as having quality ingredients and meeting A.A.F.C.O. standards. We thought we were doing well by them. Then things I was reading made me wonder if I was doing the best thing. I had a talk with my veterinarian. That discussion sparked a quest.

I spent years researching dog food: kibble vs canned vs fresh cooked vs raw diet; commercially prepared vs home made. What I've found is a tremendous amount of conflicting information, much of it presented with an agenda behind it. My veterinarian: Dr. Manes of Cedarwood Veterinary Hospital in Newport TN, helped me sort it all out.

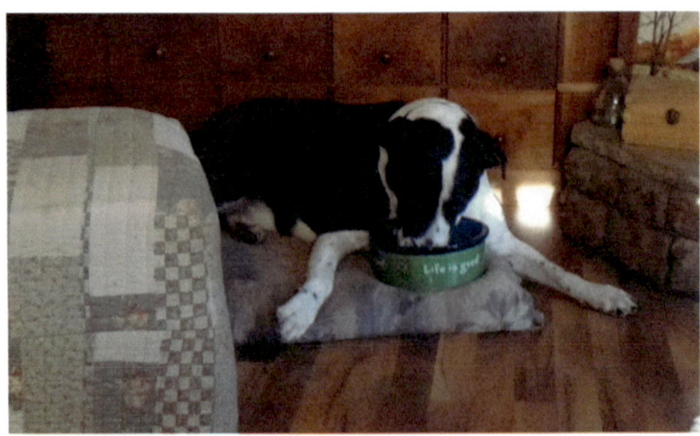

The Dog Food Dilemma

Producers of dry dog food (kibble) claim it is nutritionally complete and safe. Producers of other types of dog food claim kibble is junk food for dogs, having had all the nutritional content cooked out of it to make shelf-stable dry bits.

Canned food is supposedly better. But even a quality canned food says a dog the size of my Cochise (85 pounds) needs 6 cans of food per day to meet his minimum nutrition requirements. That's 5 pounds of food per day! And opponents say canned food is still full of bad ingredients, is high in fat, and is often recalled for contamination.

Some people insist that a raw meat diet is the only way to go: it's what a dog's digestive system was designed to handle. But recently (2019 – 2020) there have been many reports of dogs dying of heart disease caused by a diet too high in protein.

Others are pushing frozen or freeze-dried dog food as the freshest and most nutritious.

Multiple sources point out that A.A.F.C.O. (Association of American Feed Control Officials) standards for pet food are the minimum of what a pet needs in order to stay alive. Meeting these standards does not insure an animal will thrive. I want my dogs to be happy and healthy for as long as possible. So I've been researching alternatives to mass-produced commercial foods.

What I found, once I sifted out the propaganda, was enough information to fill a book! So I wrote one. I hope you enjoy it and maybe even learn a thing or two.

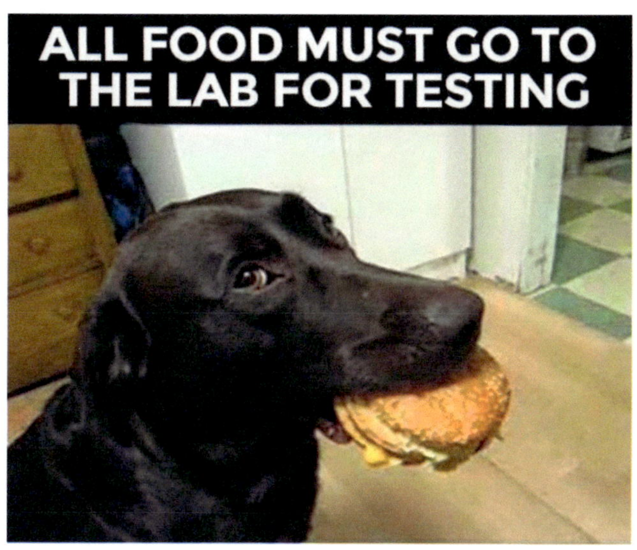

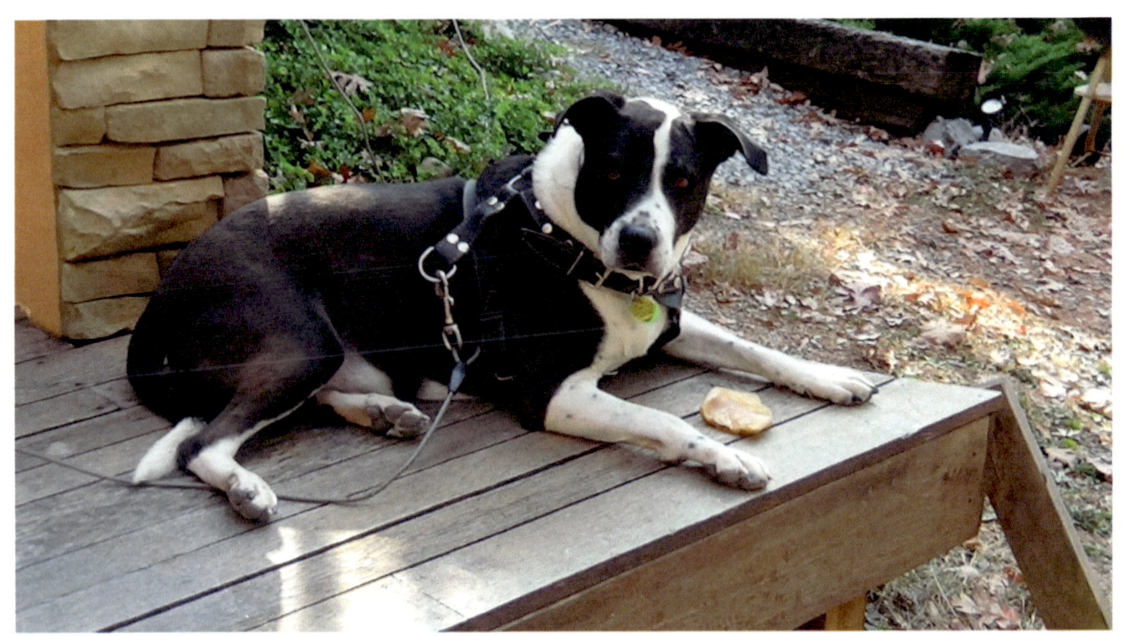

Chapter 1: Elements of Nutrition

Regardless of what type of food you eventually decide is best for you and your dog, there are some basic nutritional components to bear in mind as you evaluate your options.

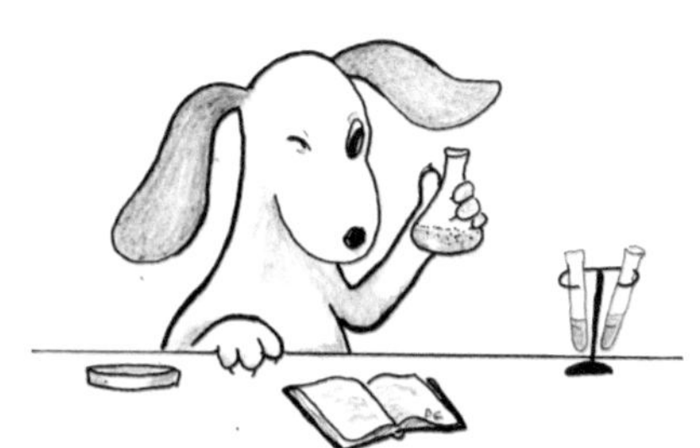

Protein

Protein is the basis of a carnivore diet. Ideally this would mean lean muscle meat, but certain organs can be mixed in as well. Heart and gizzards are more like muscle meat than typical organs. Kidney and liver are rich meats that should be used in small quantities, mixed in with the muscle meat, or they'll cause diarrhea. These are readily available in stores.

If you have access to a slaughter house, many other organs: brain, spleen, and lung, will be available at low cost. These are not normally available through typical grocery stores. Stay away from stomach and intestines as they are hard to clean properly. Beef tongue is okay, but has a tough rind that makes it difficult to work with.

Some vegetables do contain protein. Peas are about 25% protein, legumes like dried beans and chick peas are high in digestible protein as well. But a dog's gut has more trouble extracting nutrients from vegetation than a human's gut does. A vegan diet works fur humans, not for canines. However, you can add variety and cut costs by occasionally using beans, peas, legumes in your canine cookery in place of meat.

Here is a guide to common protein-rich foods from Dr. Andrea Pennington, MD

- Cottage cheese (nonfat): 1 cup has 28 grams
- Milk (nonfat): 1 cup has 10 grams
- Mozzarella cheese (nonfat): 1-ounce stick has 8 grams
- Yogurt (nonfat, sugar-free): 6-ounce carton has 5 grams
- Beef (lean): 3 ounces (cooked weight) has 25 grams
- Chicken breast: 3 ounces (cooked weight) has 25 grams
- Turkey breast: 3 ounces (cooked weight) has 25 grams
- Pork tenderloin: 3 ounces (cooked weight) has 24 grams
- Turkey ham: 4 ounces (cooked weight) has 18 grams
- Tuna: 4 ounces (water packed) has 27 grams
- Ocean-caught fish: 4 ounces (cooked weight) has 25 to 31 grams

- Shrimp, crab, lobster: 4 ounces (cooked weight) has 22 to 24 grams
- Scallops: 4 ounces (cooked weight) has 25 grams
- Lentils: 1⁄2 cup (cooked) has 9 grams
- Beans (black, pinto, etc.): 1⁄2 cup (cooked) has 7 grams

Your meat can come from any animal: beef, pork, goat, chicken, armadillo, duck, fish, anything that is lean and uncontaminated by disease or decay. (I threw that armadillo in here to see if you were paying attention. You probably don't want to try butchering an armadillo.)

Carbohydrates

Carbohydrates are an alternative energy source. Comprised primarily of starch, carbohydrates turn to sugar in the digestive process. The sugar is then used for energy. The problem with carbs is that they are short-term energy and any sugar not immediately burned off gets converted to fat and stored. Therefore, carbohydrates (or carbs) used in excess promote canine obesity and diabetes.

Carbs are found in starchy grains like corn, wheat and soy. Carrots and potatoes are starchy vegetables, thus high in carbs.

The canine digestive system (being carnivore) does not handle carbohydrates as efficiently as humans (omnivores) do. Humans can get by with eating a plant-based diet heavy on legumes for protein. Dogs cannot. Being carnivores, their systems are designed to process a meat based diet. But as with most dietary issues, the key to good health is balance.

In a healthy dog, proper proportions of carbohydrates can reduce the need for meat and provide some of the calories needed to thrive. In a diabetic or obese dog carbs should be avoided. However high fiber, low fat vegetation can be included, like legumes and nuts.

Essential Fatty Acids

Fish oils are the best source of Essential Fatty Acid (EFA). EFAs help keep the skin and coat healthy, increase energy, and speed healing of injuries. Other sources of EFAs are coconut oil, flax seed oil, and sunflower or safflower oils.

Fat

There is good fat and there is bad fat. Good fat is a concentrated source of energy, assists in the absorption of vitamins, supports the immune system as well as healthy skin and coat. Bad fat leads to obesity and pancreatitis.

The fat clinging to a cut of meat or under chicken skin is bad fat and you want to trim that away and dispose of it. Good fats come from organ meats, especially chicken and beef heart, liver, and gizzards.

Minerals

Minerals are elements found in a dog's natural food that have important effects in their bodies and need to be in balance with one another and other components of their diet.

Calcium

You know that calcium is needed for strong bones and teeth. Calcium is also important for hormone transmission, nerve function, muscle contraction, digestion, cognitive function, and blood clotting. However, too much calcium is often blamed for contributing to osteoporosis in young, rapidly growing dogs – especially large breed puppies – and can bind up certain other nutrients in your dog's diet and make them unavailable to her. Too much calcium has also been cited as a cause of canine heart problems. So we need to strike the right balance.

If you are feeding a quality commercial dog food of any form, this should be taken care of for you. The only time it would be a concern is if you add something like extra meat. Then you'll need to re-balance the formula by adding calcium. If you feed a raw meat diet or cook your own dog food it is especially important to maintain this balance. We will look at this in detail in the Home Cooking and Raw Diet sections of this book.

Copper

Copper affects the production of pigments in skin and fur, so one sign of copper deficiency is loss of pigment in the dog's coat.

Iron

Iron is an important building block of hemoglobin, which is what carries oxygen in red blood cells. Dogs need approximately 35 mg of iron daily for every pound of dried food they eat. Dietary sources for iron include:

- Liver: incorporate liver in home-made food or buy treats made out of liver.
- Lean meats: select ground beef with a high percentage of lean beef.
- Fish: serve a premium dog food made with fish or serve cooked fish in moderation like salmon or sardines. Do not serve your dog raw fish. We'll discuss why in a little while.
- Whole grains, Lima beans, and chicken.

Magnesium

Magnesium is involved in regulating hormones and guards against high urinary loss, which leads to magnesium deficiency and a risk factor for retinal damage, heart disease, and canine seizures.

Phosphorous

Phosphorous is essential for proper bone development in a dog but they don't need large amounts to be healthy. Puppies need more phosphorous (and calcium) than adult dogs because they're still growing new bone. Requirements decrease as your dog gets older and senior dogs have the smallest dietary phosphorous requirements.

Phosphorous has been shown to contribute to the progression of renal disease, so decreasing phosphorous consumption goes a long way towards slowing kidney disease's progression.

In general, foods highest in phosphorus include dairy products, fish (with bones), organ meats, and egg yolks.

Potassium

Potassium is an essential nutrient required by the body for vital functions such as pumping the heart, maintaining electrolyte balance and building muscle.

A deficiency of this important nutrient can bring about muscle weakness, abnormal heart rhythms, and fluctuations in blood pressure. However, too much potassium can also lead to dangerous heart rhythms.

Sodium

Sodium maintains the cellular environment and prevents cells from swelling or dehydrating. It is also important for maintaining proper nerve and muscle cell function.

In pet foods, meat, poultry, fish, and eggs are good sources of sodium.

The Association of American Feed Control Officials recommend that dry dog foods contain at least 0.3% sodium for support of normal growth and development. These are minimum recommended levels.

High sodium intake causes increased thirst and water consumption, but the extra sodium is excreted in the urine of dogs. Healthy dogs are able to consume higher sodium levels than found in most commercial pet foods without increased blood pressure or gain in body water. Therefore, the sodium level in commercial pet foods is not a cause for concern in healthy animals.

Zinc

Dietary zinc is important in the maintenance of skin integrity. Skin is a rapidly reproducing tissue so it has a high demand for this mineral and Zinc deficiency shows up quickly in skin and coat quality.

Vegetables

Vegetables are a great source of vitamins, minerals, and fiber. Note that excess fiber can loosen a dogs stool, so monitor him and adjust the amount of fiber you're giving accordingly.

The canine digestive tract is not as attuned to extracting nutrient from large chunks of vegetable matter like people can. To allow your dog to get essential vitamins and minerals from veggies it is recommended that you steam the veggies to break down the cellulose a bit, releasing the nutrients, then chop or mash them.

The best vegetables to use are dark green veggies like spinach and broccoli which are high in iron and vitamin C, orange veggies like sweet potato, squash or pumpkin contain beta carotene and a lot of good fiber; green beans, peas, cauliflower, and legumes (dry beans, chick peas).

Vitamins

Vitamins are an essential part of the diet of any living creature. Ideally, the needed vitamins come through their natural diet. But as domesticated animals, dogs diets are restricted. Also, many vitamins are degraded or destroyed by exposure to heat and/or water, and/or air, and/or light.

Steaming, microwaving, or using a pan or wok with a small amount of water are the preferred cooking methods. "The most vitamins are retained when there is less contact with water and a shorter cooking time", notes University of Kentucky Extension. In a Danish study, steaming broccoli for five minutes retained almost 100 percent of the water-soluble vitamins. Microwaving and stir-frying reduce vitamin loss because they cook food quickly. Avoid frying: the high heat required for frying destroys heat-sensitive vitamins. Boiling veggies is a bad practice that removes too much vitamin content, especially if you don't use the water in your recipe.

Cooking method is an especially important consideration if you choose to feed your dog a home-cooked diet. If you're hoping to provide a healthier diet, but then cook most of the nutritional value out of their food, you are defeating yourself.

The table below is from the United States Department of Agriculture and shows the effects of cooking, freezing and drying (dehydrating) on vitamin and mineral content in food.

Typical Maximum Nutrient Losses (as compared to raw food)

Vitamins	Freeze	Dry	Cook	Cook+Drain	Reheat
Vitamin A	5%	50%	25%	35%	10%
Retinol Activity Equivalent	5%	50%	25%	35%	10%
Alpha Carotene	5%	50%	25%	35%	10%
Beta Carotene	5%	50%	25%	35%	10%
Beta Cryptoxanthin	5%	50%	25%	35%	10%
Lycopene	5%	50%	25%	35%	10%
Lutein+Zeaxanthin	5%	50%	25%	35%	10%
Vitamin C	30%	80%	50%	75%	50%
Thiamin	5%	30%	55%	70%	40%
Riboflavin	0%	10%	25%	45%	5%
Niacin	0%	10%	40%	55%	5%
Vitamin B6	0%	10%	50%	65%	45%
Folate	5%	50%	70%	75%	30%
Food Folate	5%	50%	70%	75%	30%
Folic Acid	5%	50%	70%	75%	30%
Vitamin B12	0%	0%	45%	50%	45%
Minerals	**Freeze**	**Dry**	**Cook**	**Cook+Drain**	**Reheat**
Calcium	5%	0%	20%	25%	0%
Iron	0%	0%	35%	40%	0%
Magnesium	0%	0%	25%	40%	0%
Phosphorus	0%	0%	25%	35%	0%
Potassium	10%	0%	30%	70%	0%
Sodium	0%	0%	25%	55%	0%
Zinc	0%	0%	25%	25%	0%
Copper	10%	0%	40%	45%	0%

Chapter 2: Dry Dog Food

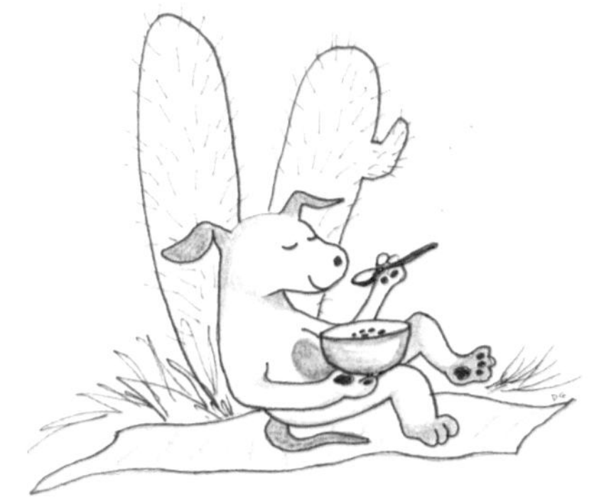

Dry dog food is the most common means of feeding a dog. There are hundreds of brands available to choose from and they cover the whole spectrum from cheap, store-brand kibble to specialty, gourmet dry food. Choosing from among this array of possibilities is a daunting task.

DogFoodAdvosor.com says, "The biggest mistakes we see people make when shopping for dog food are that they fail to check the label for the A.A.F.C.O. statement, and never buy any dog food that's not suitable for your dog's stage of life. For example, a puppy should NEVER be fed a food designed for an adult dog." A dog should stay on puppy food for their first full year of life to insure proper bone and muscle development. Likewise, food designed for a young adult dog is too high in calories for a senior dog and will lead to obesity.

Here are some pointers of what to look for (or look out for) when reading the label on a bag of dog food.

Assessing a dry dog food

It is not practical to try to list the entire database of information used by dog food rating sites. In the following section I will point out the major items that you are likely to encounter and explain what they mean. With this knowledge you can evaluate most dry dog food labels.

Where is it made?

To start with: do not feed your dog Chinese-made store-brand kibble. China is particularly notorious for using fillers like melamine in their pet foods to boost profits. Some of these have proven to be poisonous and many animals have died. Law suits have been filed, but because the manufacturer is in a foreign country, compliance with our food standards is voluntary and legal action cannot be taken against them. We can pressure American distributors to discontinue offering deadly brands, but the manufacturer just changes the brand name and keeps on selling it.

While you can avoid Chinese-made foods, you cannot so easily tell if the ingredients used in a non-Chinese made dog food aren’t sourced from China. Even top brands like Merrick have been sued after their product killed dogs because of ingredients originating from China. *Dogs Naturally Magazine* reported, "In 2007, 150 major brands of pet foods were recalled after several thousand dogs and cats died. The FDA reported these recalls were the consequence of combining melamine and cyanuric acid, which reacted in the pets eating these foods, causing sudden, complete kidney failure."

It is, therefore, incumbent upon the buyer to be aware of any risks by researching the brands available. I will not recommend one brand over another, but I will say that I've trusted **www.DogFoodAdvisor.com** for analysis and reviews as well as notification of recalls. Check out their web site, peruse their listing of top-rated brands. Find one that is available to you and suits your budget.

What's in it?

Read the label on a potential dog food carefully, and not just the front of the bag. Focus on the back of the bag. The front of the bag tends to be pure marketing: attractive pictures, a catchy name, and statements concerning its quality and desirability – which, by the way, are not verified for truthfulness by the FDA because this is not for human consumption. Basically, pet food manufacturers can make any claim they want in their promotional content and get away with even blatant lies. It's up to you to verify these claims.

The back label lists ingredients and nutrition testing results. These are supposed to be accurate, but even here there are ways to cheat so it looks better than it is. Ingredients are to be listed in decreasing order of content. Whatever is listed first is the primary component, what's listed next is the next largest part of the formula, etcetera. You want your dog's food to be made primarily of wholesome, nutritious food. For a dog, that should be some kind of real meat.

Meat and meat derivatives

Because dogs are carnivores, they need a high protein diet. That means meat. However, if the first listed ingredient is "Meat", do not rejoice. What kind of meat?

A generic name like this is an attempt to hide the true nature of this ingredient. If the front of the bag says something like, "Crunchy Beef Bits" but the back of the bag says, "meat", run away! Any beef flavor this kibble contains will be artificial.

When the front of the bag says, "beef", "pork", "lamb", "venison", "buffalo", "chicken", "turkey", "duck" or "salmon" that meat should be the first ingredient listed.

If the first ingredient is "beef byproducts", put the bag down and look for another one. Byproducts are the trash left over from the butchering process: lips and butt-holes; as some say. There may be a place for this stuff, but that's definitely not the top slot on the ingredients list.

Beef (pork, lamb, chicken, etc) **meal** is okay. Beef and bone meal, as stated by A.A.F.C.O., is the rendered product from beef tissues, including bone, exclusive of any added blood, hair, hoof, horn, hide trimmings, manure, stomach and rumen contents, (byproducts) except in such amounts as may occur unavoidably in good processing practices.

Basically meat meal is dehydrated meat, or a meat concentrate. It is actually a more protein-dense ingredient (most meat meal contains nearly 300% more protein by volume than fresh meat) because the water has been removed. Remember that the label lists raw ingredients by volume, so if raw meat is used it will end up being a smaller volume in the cooked kibble because the water content is driven out. Raw chicken, for example, is about 80% water. After processing, most of that moisture is lost, reducing the meat content to just a small fraction of its original weight. But there is no way to get around that, so some manufacturers add meat meal as well as the primary meat to insure the required protein content. Note: I used the term "meat meal" as a broad spectrum label in this discussion, you do not want to see "Meat meal" as an ingredient any more than you want to see "Meat" as an ingredient. Beef meal, chicken meal, duck meal, etcetera are fine. "Meat meal" is highly questionable.

Chicken fat is obtained while rendering chicken in a process similar to making soup in which the fat itself is skimmed from the surface of the liquid. This is high in linoleic acid, an omega-6 fatty acid essential for life. It doesn't sound very appetizing, but chicken fat is actually a quality ingredient in dog food, as long as it's further down the list, and your dog does not have kidney issues.

Grains

Corn, wheat, and soy have only one purpose in dog food: filler. Some manufacturers use these as a calorie source because they are starchy: the carbohydrates convert to sugar, the sugar gives a dog energy. It also makes them fat and promotes diabetes. Any kibble that lists corn, wheat, or soy as the first ingredient gets an automatic fail. I personally recommend passing on any kibble that lists any grain in the first three ingredients. Dogs need protein, not carbs (refer to MEAT above).

That said, there is a place in a dog kibble formula for healthy grain. White rice is okay, brown rice is better. Oats are great, barley, and sorghum are good: somewhere down the list of ingredients, not at the top. These grains add fiber and trace minerals. Oatmeal is naturally rich in B-vitamins. Ground flax seed is one of the best plant-based sources of omega-3 fatty acids and is rich in soluble fiber.

People call quinoa (pronounced "keen-whah") a grain, but it's actually a seed — one that originated thousands of years ago in the Andes Mountains. Treasured because of its nutritive value (more protein than any other grain or seed), quinoa is a flowering plant in the amaranth family (botanically related to spinach and amaranth) grown as a grain crop for its edible seeds. Quinoa is the only food of vegetable origin that provides all the essential amino acids, trace elements and vitamins, equating its protein quality to that of milk. It is gluten-free. Its grains are highly nutritious, surpassing cereals, such as wheat, corn, rice, and oats, in biological value and nutritional quality. After harvest, the seeds are processed to remove the bitter-tasting outer seed coat.

Whole grains (including the hulls and germ of the kernel) are usually best – but rarely used in commercial dog food. Grain flour and meal are the cast-offs of milling these grains for human use and are more often what ends up in mass-produced pet food. In a certain sense, this is good because a study found the carbohydrates in grain are more digestible for dogs when the grain is ground into flour. Barley flour is five times more digestible in dogs than whole barley, and rice flour is ten times more digestible than whole rice (Bednar et al, 2000).

Vegetables

Sweet potatoes are a gluten-free source of complex carbohydrates in a dog food. They are naturally rich in dietary fiber and beta carotene. Squash and pumpkin are almost as good.

Peas are a quality source of carbohydrates. Plus (like all legumes) they're rich in natural fiber. Peas contain about 25% protein, a factor to consider when judging the actual meat content of this dog food.

Potatoes can be considered a gluten-free source of digestible carbohydrates, but are of only modest nutritional value to a dog.

Any dark green vegetable (spinach, broccoli, collards, etc) is rich in vitamins and minerals in their natural state but these are reduced or destroyed by high-temperature cooking (see Chapter 1).

Corn: see Grains above.

Illicit Additives

When you get down the list of ingredients you start seeing things with unpronounceable names. Sometimes this is bad, but sometimes these are synthesized vitamins and oils. You can do an internet search on each of these to find out what they do and if they are good or bad. Of course, good and bad are subjective depending on how much of a purist one is.

We should always be disappointed to find **artificial coloring** in any pet food. Coloring is used to make the product more appealing … to humans. Do you really think your dog cares what color his food is?

You do not want to see artificial preservatives, like BHA, BHT, or ethoxyquin. Natural preservatives such as tocopherols (compounds with vitamin E), vitamin C, and rosemary extract are better. Natural preservatives do not preserve dog foods as long as artificial preservatives, so owners should always check the label's "best by" date.

Your dog's food should be flavored well enough with healthy meats and fats to be enticing to him. There should be no need for any **artificial flavors**.

Like us, dogs have a taste for sweets. Corn syrup, sucrose, ammoniated glycyrrhizin, and other sweeteners are sometimes added to low-quality foods to make them more appealing to your dog. Excessive dietary sugar causes health problems, including obesity and diabetes, in dogs. Avoid foods with excessive sweeteners and anything with Xylitol in it as this is poisonous to dogs.

Nutritional Content

The thing I find most worrisome about dry kibble is that even the best brands, which use quality ingredients, cook their product at such high heat as to render all that fresh food into small brown pebbles. These store well and are convenient to feed, but how much nutrition is left after such rigorous processing? I know from cooking food for my family that high heat kills many vitamins and we are encouraged to prepare our food at the lowest temperature that will do the job. Can it be any less so for dog food? This is what spurred my consult with Dr. Manes.

Expecting an animal to thrive on a diet of commercial kibble is like people eating nothing but box meals and fast food. They can (and do) survive, but will not be among the healthiest people you know and many of their health issues are directly related to their diet.

Amending a Kibble Diet

Later I will discuss alternative diets, including home cooked "stew" for dogs and raw meat diets. However, taking the leap into free-style home-prepared dog food may not be something you can do at this point in your life. Maybe you don't cook. If you can't or don't cook for your own family, expecting you to cook for your dog is pointless. If you do not have the time, space, or skills to cook for your dog, what can you do to make her diet more healthy? There are a number of things you can do to boost nutrition content of dry kibble with minimal fuss.

When using an amendment, do remember to decrease the amount of commercial food your dog gets so you don't increase the total number of calories you feed your dog. This can lead to unhealthy weight gain. Also, limit the amount of fresh food you add to about 25 percent of total calories consumed, and rotate your additions to provide a better balanced over-all diet and prevent onset of food allergies.

Start with Quality Kibble

As I have said above, despite what the kibble manufacturers tell you, dry kibble alone is not a healthful diet. Some are better than others, so find a good one and go from there.

Canned Fish

Adding canned tuna, mackerel, sardines packed in water (not oil or mustard), or especially salmon, to your dog's kibble is a good way to add the omega-3 fatty acids EPA and DHA. These essential fatty acids help heal sore, flaky, damaged, or itchy skin. This is because Omega-3 fats found in fish oil help to reduce inflammation, which can lessen the intensity of many allergies. Omega-3 fats can also reduce a dog's reaction to pollen and other common allergy triggers found in the environment. These also help regulate the immune system. This is helpful for dogs with allergies, arthritis, and autoimmune disease. DHA is also good for brain health, which can benefit both puppies and senior dogs.

One small canned sardine (2 tsp of canned tuna, mackerel, or salmon) provides about 25 calories and 175 mg of omega-3 fatty acids, a good amount for a dog of 20 pounds or less. Give larger dogs proportionately more. An 80 pound dog can have 4 small sardines or 8 tsp (roughly 2½ Tbsp) of canned or fresh fish.

Cooking raw fish is healthier but more trouble. Feeding your dog raw fish opens them up to potential parasite infestation unless you freeze the fish for at least a week then thaw and feed.

Egg

Fresh eggs are great for dogs, are inexpensive, and easy to feed. Eggs offer a combination of high-quality protein and good fat along with a variety of vitamins and minerals.

Egg whites are more easily digested when cooked, but yolks retain more nutritional value if fed raw. Most dogs have no trouble with bacteria in raw eggs, but it's safer to feed soft-cooked or scrambled eggs as a compromise to raw yolk.

One large egg provides around 70 calories; this amount is fine for medium-sized (30 pounds and larger) dogs, but smaller dogs would do better with an egg every other day (or less). Remember to reduce the kibble proportionately.

Do not include the shell when you feed your dog an egg and kibble. Combining crushed egg shell and kibble will provide far more calcium than your dog needs. Too much calcium can be harmful to large-breed puppies and binds other minerals in your dog's food, making them less available to your dog.

Yogurt

The probiotics (beneficial bacteria) in yogurt provide healthful benefits to all dogs, especially to dogs with digestive problems. Use yogurt with live, active cultures. Stick to low-fat or nonfat plain yogurt as your dog does not need the sugar in the flavored varieties nor the added fat of regular yogurt.

Low-fat yogurt provides fewer than 20 calories per ounce, so even small dogs can enjoy a spoonful of yogurt on their kibble without concern about reducing the food portion.

Fruits and Vegetables

Blueberries are chock full of antioxidants. Other good fruits to feed include bananas, apples, papaya, and melon. Some dogs like oranges. Don't include the pits. Avoid grapes and raisins which can cause kidney failure in dogs when eaten in quantity. Fruits are high in sugar, so they add to calorie counts, reduce kibble accordingly.

- 1 Apple: 81 calories, 21 carbs
- 1 avg Banana: 105 calories, 27 carbs
- ½ cup fresh Blueberries: 41 calories, 10 carbs
- 1/10 Cantaloupe: 19 calories, 9 carbs
- 1/10 Honeydew: 46 calories, 12 carbs
- 1 Orange: 65 calories, 16 carbs
- ½ Papaya: 27 calories, 7 carbs

- 1 Peach: 37 calories, 10 carbs
- 1 med Pear: 98 calories, 25 carbs
- 1 Tomato: 26 calories, 6 carbs
- 1 cherry tomato: 3 calories, 1 carb

Leafy green vegetables are a better choice for adding to kibble than starchy foods like potatoes. Vegetables are more nutritious when fed steamed to release their nutrients; but raw veggies such as carrots, zucchini slices, and frozen peas or green beans, make great low-calorie snacks. Non-starchy vegetables can be included in your dog's meals without adding significant calories.

Canned pumpkin (straight pumpkin not pie mix), squash, and sweet potato are high in fiber and are great for promoting regularity. Naturally, using these fresh and steaming, or microwaving them, is better than canned; but if you're in a rush canned will do. Just watch the sodium content in anything canned.

Cruciferous veggies, like broccoli, Brussel sprouts, cabbage, and cauliflower often cause an increase in gas and flatulence. Use with caution or lots of ventilation!

Meat

Muscle meat: be it from chicken, turkey, duck, deer, or lean beef; ground, shredded, or cut in small chunks (to avoid choking) is a great source of protein.

Organ Meat, such as liver, spleen or kidney, should be fed in small amounts because it is rich and can lead to diarrhea but is loaded with beneficial nutrients. Organ meats like hearts and gizzards are nutritionally more like muscle meats and can be fed in greater quantity.

Mixing a small portion of organ meat in with a larger portion of muscle meat is a good way to get the benefits of both types of meat without risking gastric upset. This is easy to do if you grind the meat. Grinding also allows you to add calcium right into the mix.

When adding meat to kibble, add 1/2 tsp. ground eggshell or 1,000 mg calcium powder per pound of meat to maintain the proper calcium/phosphorus ratio. Adding calcium is not necessary if the added meat is only a small portion such as a sprinkling of cubes over the kibble. If meat is 25% of the meal or more, add the proper amount of calcium.

Grains

Don't do this. Commercial dog kibble is high in carbohydrate-rich grains so there is no advantage to adding grains by way of cooked oatmeal, rice, or barley cereal. All you will do is boost the carbs, which turn to sugar, and throw the caloric count out of whack. Grains are helpful in making a full meal dog food, but we will discuss that in the next chapter.

Bone Broth

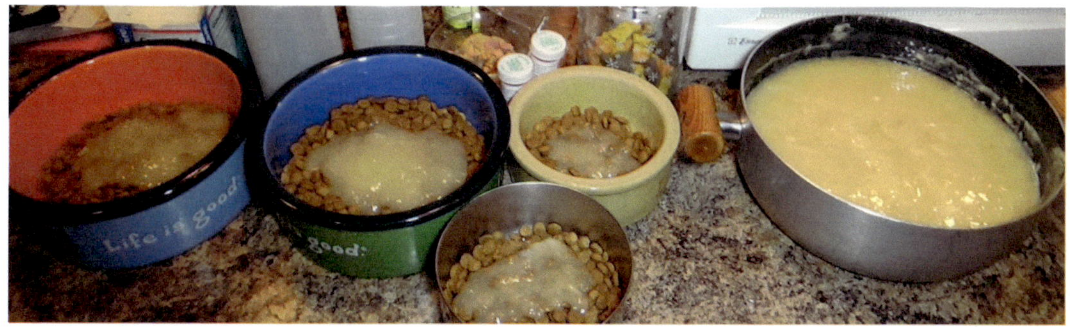

Bone broth has been traditionally used to treat leaky gut and digestive issues, but has many health benefits. It benefits dogs with allergies and food sensitivities, as it is an immune system booster, while also supporting good joint health.

Bone broth is rich in many nutrients, especially amino acids such as arginine, glycine, glutamine and proline. Bone broth also acts as a superior joint supplement, as it contains gelatin (the breakdown of collagen), glucosamine, and chondroitin that support good joint health.

Protein rich bone broth contains vitamin C, vitamin D, vitamin K, iron, thiamin, potassium, calcium, silicon, sulfer, magnesium, glucosamine, phosphorus, trace minerals, and glucosamine chondroitin sulfates.

It's easy to make too – even if you don't normally cook. If you have a crock pot you can make bone broth. I'll cover the process in detail in Chapter 5, but basically you just simmer meat bones in water for 8 to 24 hours. If you can boil water you can make bone broth.

For healthy dogs, a dollop of bone broth over kibble once a day is an excellent whole food multivitamin. Dogs 80 to 100 pounds need ½ cup (4 ounces) of bone broth per day. Split that if you feed twice a day. Doing a little math: a dog 60 pounds to 80 would get ¾ cup (or 6 oz.) per day, 40 to 60 pounds: ½ cup (4 oz.), 20 to 40 pounds: ¼ cup (2 oz.) and dogs 20 pounds and under only need an ounce (2 Tbsp) or so per day. Remember: if you feed twice a day: either split these amounts or add the full amount to only one meal.

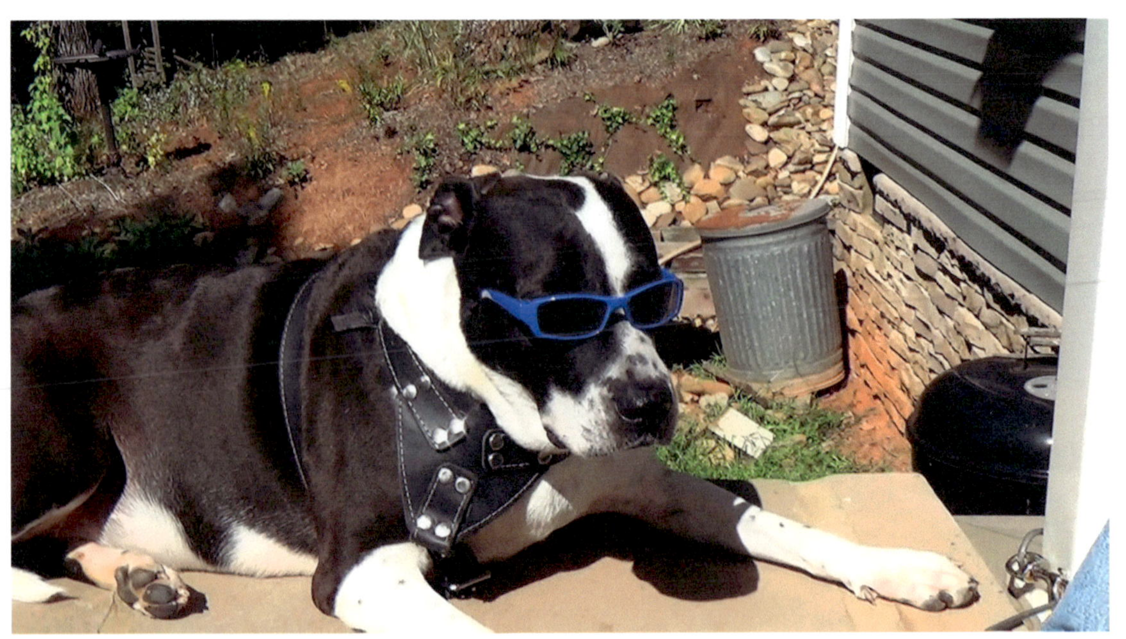

Chapter 3: Home-Cooking For Your Dog

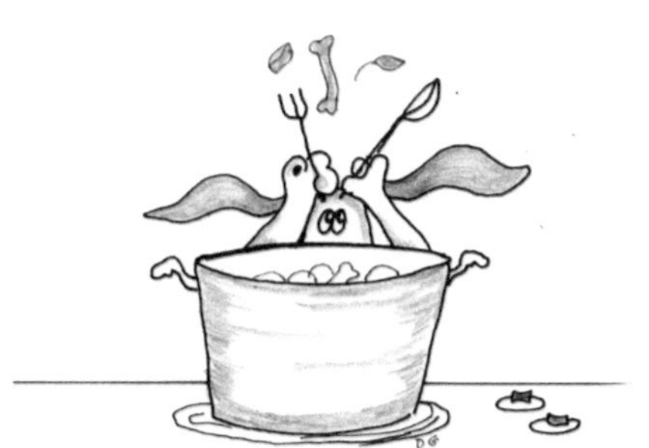

Much of the confusion about home cooked dog food comes from the fact that much of the information available on-line is presented by "nutritionists" who want the reader to pay them to design meal plans and recipes tailored to their dog's breed, age, health, and environment. This is a good thing for those who can afford it. One dog's dietary needs will not necessarily fit those of a different dog: large, small; young and active, old and sedentary; each have different nutritional needs. Even the breed can have an effect: a Husky will need a different balance than a Basset. For those of us who can't afford such a service, I kept digging to attain the basic information needed to do it right.

The Veterinarian's View

Doctor Sandra Manes DVM has always been honest with me as well as being well versed in everything we've needed. We had a long discussion. I won't relate it all, but the distillation is that, while she will not denigrate anyone for feeding their dog a commercial diet – unless the dog's health issues are a result of that diet – she does not consider any commercially produced pet food to be completely safe or as nutritionally complete as a home-cooked dog food diet. If asked (and I asked) she says, “Always know the source of your food, and your pet’s food.” and recommends a home-cooked diet. Dr. Sandra has been invaluable in guiding me as I wrote this book, and in obtaining veterinarian level medical information.

Benefits of Home-Made Dog Food

By personally selecting the ingredients in your dog’s food, especially if your dog has allergies, you can be sure to avoid problematic ingredients and you know how your dog’s food is prepared.

- You can choose the quality of the food you use. Choose food from a local farmer, farmer’s market, grocery store, or use a bulk source. You can use certified organic, free-range, grass fed meat if that’s important to you. Or not.

- Making food for your dog is no more difficult than making food for your family but it is far more nutritious than commercial dog food.
- Even the pickiest dog loves to eat "people food" she saw (and smelled) you prepare in your own kitchen.
- Dogs who have been fed lesser quality commercial foods will develop smaller, more compact stools once the useless grain fillers (corn, soy, wheat) have been removed from their diet.
- Dogs are more likely to be well-muscled and lean on a home-made dog food diet, according to people who feed this kind of diet.
- Other benefits include good skin, good breath, clean teeth, and less doggy odor.

The Down-Side

Time and effort are the biggest drawback. It takes time to cook the food, but also to shop for it.

Time, effort and perhaps money spent finding suitable recipes to follow – attaining the right balance of protein, starch, vitamins, and various minerals is important.

To reduce time and effort, you'll want to make up your home-made dog food in pretty large batches. That means carving out room in your fridge or freezer (or both) to store the unused portion.

Considerations

So, what do you need to consider when planning to create home-made dog food? NOTE: as you look over these specifications, do not obsess over exact formulations or percentages for each and every batch. The goal – as in your own food – is to produce a balanced diet over the long haul.

Carnivore vs Omnivore

Don't make the mistake of feeding your dog whatever you eat. Human physiology is not the same as that of canines. We are omnivores and are capable of eating many things that are useless or even toxic to dogs. Carnivores also require different balances of nutrients than we do.

Raw or Cooked?

There is a heated debate among pet food “experts” about whether dogs – being descended from wolves – should be fed a raw meat diet (including the bones) like their ancestors. It's of little concern to me personally because if I put a hunk of raw meat in front of Blondie or Cochise, they look at me with skepticism, "You forgot to cook that." So my wolf descendants are a bit too civilized for raw diet to even enter the discussion. I will, however, cover the topic of raw dog food, home made and commercially available, in Chapter 5.

When cooking vegetables, be careful not to destroy the vitamin content. All the B vitamins are sensitive to heat, but thiamine, also known as vitamin B-1, and folic acid, or vitamin B-12, are the most unstable and likely to be destroyed by cooking and improper storage, according to University of Kentucky Extension Service. In a study published in the November 2010 issue of the "Journal of the Pakistan Medical Association," boiling milk for 15 minutes caused depletion of vitamins B-1, B-2, B-3, B-6 and folate by 24 to 36 percent. The earlier Danish study that evaluated the effect of boiling on vitamin C content also studied how the B vitamins in broccoli fared. After five minutes of boiling, between 45 and 64 percent of the vitamin B-6 and folate in broccoli disappeared.

Boiling vegetables in water that is drained off and discarded also discards much of the nutrient. It is better to steam or microwave vegetables to soften them. If you must boil, keep the liquid and use it for moisture in the recipe. For more on cooking vegetables for maximum food value, see Chapter 1.

Home-Made Dog Food Ingredients

The foundation of any healthy diet is variety. To avoid developing food allergies, you want to vary the specific ingredients used so each batch is not just like the last.

Your dog needs protein from animal meat, seafood, dairy, or eggs; fat from meat or oil; and some carbohydrates from good grains or starchy vegetables. He also needs calcium from dairy, calcium citrate, or an ingredient such as pulverized egg shells, and essential fatty acids from certain plant oils, egg yolks, or oatmeal.

In general, dog food should be 1/3 protein (from meat, eggs, or dairy products) and 2/3 vegetables and wholesome grain. Many dog food recipes fall short in certain nutrients, especially iron (liver, broccoli, spinach), copper (shellfish, whole grains, beans, nuts, potatoes), calcium (calcium citrate, cheese, yogurt), and zinc (meat, sea food, and liver). When you create a home-made dog food recipe, choose foods that are high in these elements, and use ingredients in the following proportions:

Protein (30%)

- Organ meats such as liver and kidneys (small amounts mixed with muscle meat)
- Muscle meat or fish
- Dairy such as yogurt, goat milk, and low-fat cheese
- Eggs: as an ingredient or soft-scrambled and laid on top.

Vegetables (40%)

- Sweet potato or squash are high in fiber to promote regularity
- Potatoes a source of starch
- Peas and Legumes such as chick peas and dry beans. Peas also provide protein
- Green veggies like broccoli and spinach are high in iron and vitamin C

Steam and mash or chop (a food processor works well) vegetables so your dog can get the nutrients from them. Most raw veggies are indigestible by dogs because their gut cannot break down cellulose.

Healthy grains (30%)

Like vegetables, gains need to be steamed and mashed or ground into flour prior to cooking to make the nutrients available to your dog's digestive system. If you boil grains, retain the fluid and use it for moisture as you make your stew.

- brown rice
- oatmeal
- barley
- sorghum
- amaranth
- quinoa
- couscous
- bulgar
- ground flax seed is one of the best plant-based sources of omega-3 oil.

In all cases, whole grain (meaning with hull and germ intact) is preferred for maximum fiber and nutrient content, even if the grain is then ground into meal or flour.

Fruits

Small amounts of apple, orange, peach, papaya, banana, etc. as a treat can be beneficial but use sparingly because of their sugar content (see the chart in Chapter 1).

Calcium

You know that calcium is needed for strong bones and teeth. Calcium is also important for hormone transmission, nerve function, muscle contraction, digestion, cognitive function, and blood clotting. However, too much calcium is often blamed for contributing to osteoporosis in young, rapidly growing dogs – especially large breed puppies – and can bind up certain other nutrients in your dog's diet and make them unavailable to her. Too much calcium has been cited as a cause of canine heart problems. On the other hand, overly high amounts of calories and protein can add to large breed puppy skeletal issues, so we need to strike the right balance.

The calcium in a dog's food should be in the correct proportion to the phosphorus the dog gets, so it will depend on the amount of meat the dogs eats. Dogs who eat meat with bones don't have to worry about this calcium to phosphorus ratio because the calcium is in the bones. When people cook for their dogs there are generally few bones in the food so they have to add calcium at a rate of 1000 mg of calcium per pound of meat.

Adding calcium can be done with bone meal, calcium citrate, or powdered egg shell. Do not count the calcium native to the dairy food in your dog's diet. Egg shell is calcium carbonate and is the least absorbable by a dog but is the most potent source. Calcium citrate is a supplement available from any source that sells vitamins. For convenience, buy the 1000 mg capsules that can be opened to release the powder within. Bone meal is just what it sounds like, ground bone. Just be sure to get the kind made for consumption, NOT the bone meal sold for use in a garden.

For each pound of raw meat add 1000 mg of calcium citrate, or ½ Tbsp of bone meal, or ½ teaspoon powdered egg shell.

If you grind bones to get a calcium supplement, use raw bones: don't cook them. Cooking, especially boiling, seriously depletes the calcium content.

Controversy

Nutritionists disagree when it comes to supplemental calcium sources (see below). Some say you must reduce your primary calcium source if you use any of these supplemental sources so you don't throw the calcium/phosphorous ratio out of whack, others insist these supplemental sources provide only traces that won't matter all that much. Personally, I agree with the latter: including spinach or broccoli in your stew does not require you to recalculate your calcium addition. If you are making a stew that uses salmon or tuna as the primary meat, which are high in calcium, then yes: consider that and reduce the added calcium accordingly. But other meats are less of a concern. Bearing that in mind, here are some supplemental calcium sources:

Yogurt, milk, and cheese (a lot of dogs prefer the taste of cottage cheese, it is also easier to digest) are supplemental sources of calcium but also rate high in fat. Yogurt is good for your pet, and provides him with natural probiotics, but it should not be used as a primary source of calcium.

Salmon, tuna, sardines, and trout are rich in calcium. Cook the fish before giving it to your pet. Raw fish may be upsetting for your pet's stomach and may also contain disease-causing bacteria or parasites (worms that infest your dog's muscle tissue – see chapter 5 for details).

Other sources of calcium are spinach, beans, sweet potato, whole wheat or broccoli.

Ingredients to Avoid

- Avocado
- Grapes and raisins
- Any fruit pits or seeds (many contain cyanide)
- Chocolate
- Macadamia nuts and walnuts
- Meat fat (causes pancreatitis)
- Mushrooms
- Mustard seeds
- Onions and onion powder
- Garlic (raw, cooked, or powdered)
- Uncooked yeast dough
- Sugar (leads to obesity and diabetes)
- Any food containing the sweetener Xylitol (fine for people, poisonous to dogs)

And of course items like coffee grounds, tea, and alcohol should be kept away from pets. For more information, please see the ASPCA's Animal Poison Control Center website at https://www.aspca.org/pet-care/animal-poison-control

How Much To Feed?

When doling out home-cooked dog food, plan on feeding your dog 2% to 3% percent of his ideal body weight per day, depending on activity level. Divide that amount in two if you feed him a morning and evening meal. Recipes are included in Chapter 6. Like any food, adjust that for the dog's activity level: a dog who lies around will need less food than one who runs and plays a lot.

For example: Cochise weights 85 pounds, he's muscular and active, so he needs 2.5 pounds of home-made dog food per day. Since he gets fed twice a day, each meal will be 1¼ pounds of food. If it's been rainy or he's being especially lazy, he'll get 1 pound of food per meal.

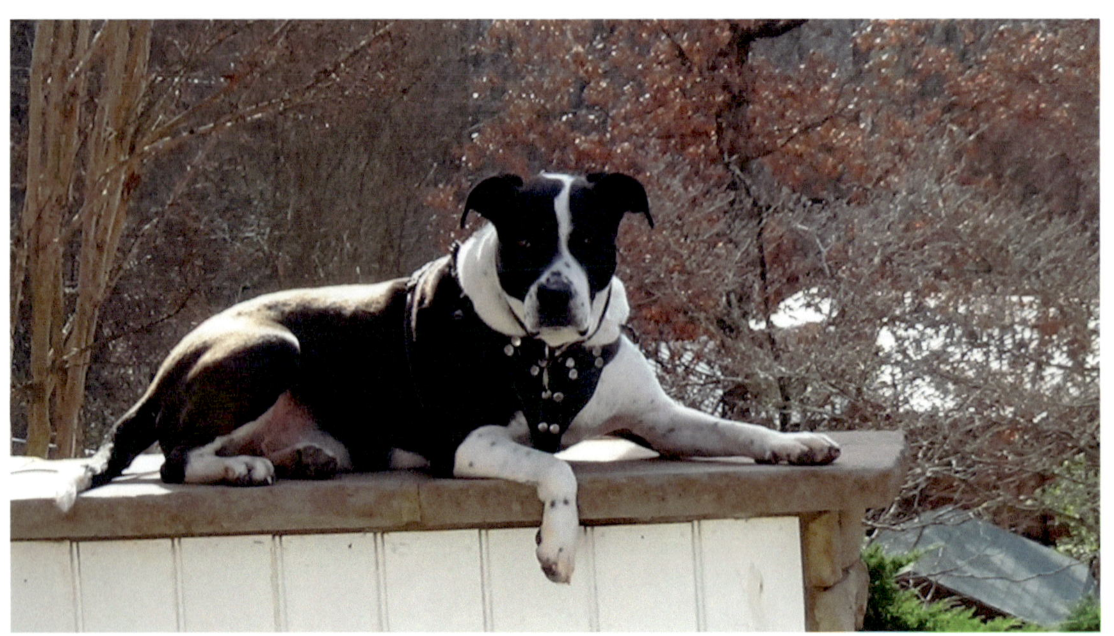

Chapter 4: Refrigerated and Freeze-Dried

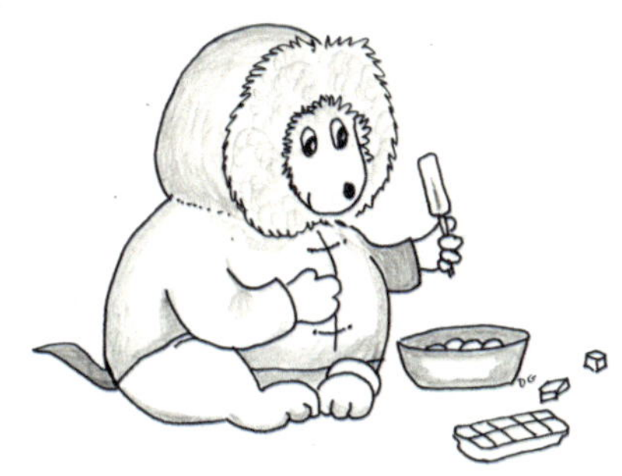

There are a number of brands of dog food that you can find in a refrigerator case in your grocery store. The only one I have personally tried is Freshpet.

This comes in a plastic tube (like breakfast sausage does) and has the consistency of braunschweiger. As you can see, there are bits of vegetables embedded in the meat pate'. This was helpful in enticing a foster dog who had had surgery to eat. It worked too: he loved it.

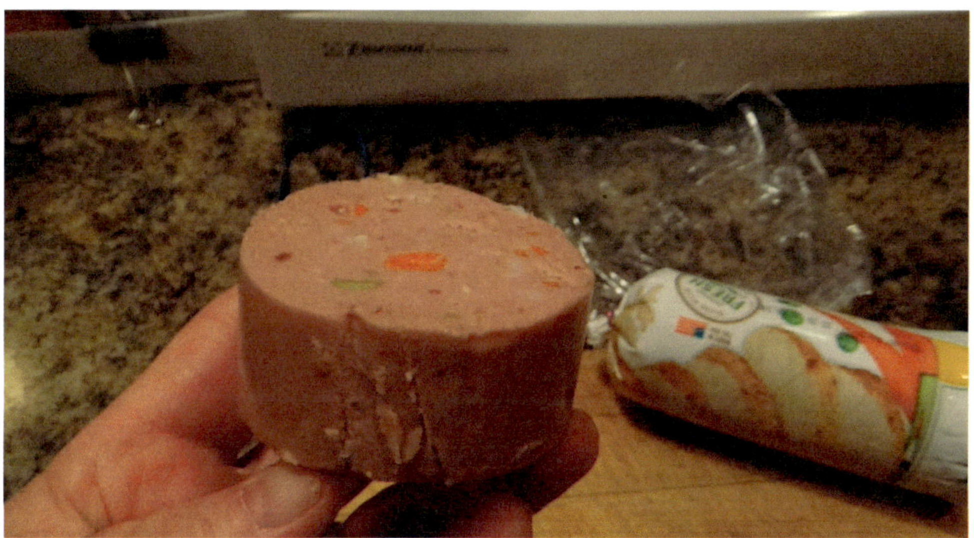

Freshpet states, "The only ingredients we're interested in are the best ingredients we can find. Every recipe we make starts with 100% farm-raised chicken, beef or fish, and all-natural fruits and veggies grown right here in the USA. Freshpet Kitchens are registered with APHIS and the FDA. We cook our meals according to FDA and USDA standards. And all of our meals undergo over 20 quality and safety tests before leaving our Kitchens." They offer a variety of flavors in rolls of 1 pound, 1.5 pound and 4 pounds. Their web site says some flavors and sizes are "*Exclusively available at Costco Stores*". Our local Food City store carries the 1.5 pound tubes in several flavors for $5.49 (at time of publication). Prices are provided ONLY for comparisons, they will change with time. This brand also offers cups of stew and dry food, but I haven't tried those.

DogFoodAdvisor.com lists the Freshpet turkey rolled dog food and gives it a 3.5 (out of 5) star rating. Their main objection is, "However, with 58% of the total calories in our example coming from fat versus just 27% from protein, some recipes may not be suitable for every animal. In addition, this same finding also prevents us from awarding the brand a higher rating."

Custom Cookery

During the research and writing of this book, I noticed an explosion in the number of services that offer custom designed, fresh delivered dog food. They all offer to have a nutritionist create recipes specifically for your dog (you fill out an on-line form with details of your dog and its lifestyle), cooked by their chef (some claim Master Chef), and delivered to your home periodically. Some come in individual serving pouches or tubs, some come in plastic pouches that you split into three or four meals.

Because I've encountered so many of these, I assume the popularity is increasing. Generally, pricing is not discussed until after you've filled out their information form. I obtained pricing from Farmer's Dog (a full custom service) at $7.75 per meal, but they do offer discounts to regular customers when they reorder. Another brand also offers a half-dozen "standard recipes" which sold for $10.50 per 16 ounce serving. That will get you into the ball-park, the more customized a service is the higher the price will be. For those who desire a quality diet for their dog but don't cook their own meals, much less for their pet, this could be a viable option. All brands tout customized nutrition, highest quality ingredients, individual servings of fresh food delivered to your door. Most offer free delivery – which just means the delivery cost is factored into their food price. Just do your homework and research several services to be sure their customers are happy with the service and food being delivered. Also make sure they offer a balanced diet that does not fall into any of the traps of those "trendy" diets.

Dehydrated Dog Food

There are a number of brands that offer air-dried or freeze-dried dog food. The makers claim that their special process retains the vitamins and minerals that are normally processed out of dog food when turned into kibble.

Customer comments on dried dog food which contain vegetables and grain as well as meat state that what you get after hydration bears no resemblance to fresh, raw meat. That is not surprising, however, since the dog food combines meat with fresh fruits and vegetables, these would have to be ground up together and formed into nuggets or strips before drying. The strips come out like jerky.

There are single ingredient meat products (photo below) that are a bag of freeze-dried meat chunks, and these do reconstitute to be meat, or can be fed dried as a treat. My dogs love the liver lumps, the chicken is pretty powdery when fed dry. They congregate around the water bowl when I give mine the chicken as it comes out of the bag. But when reconstituted it becomes white meat chicken!

There is also a form of dried raw meat that comes as pellets to be added as a topper to regular kibble without hydration.

Freeze drying is a low temperature dehydration process which involves rapidly freezing the product, lowering pressure (inducing partial vacuum), then removing the ice by sublimation. This is in contrast to dehydration by most conventional methods that evaporate water using heat. Freeze drying results in a high quality product because of the low temperature used in processing. The original shape of the product is maintained and quality of the rehydrated product is excellent.

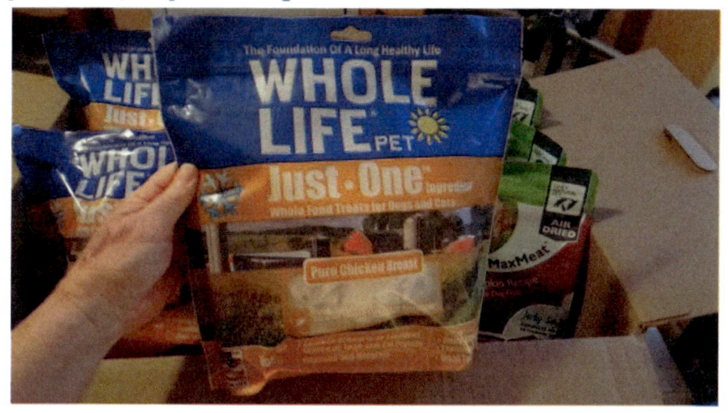

This product is delivered as single ingredient freeze-dried chunks or nuggets in a vacuum sealed bag. They are shelf-stable as long as they are kept dry. You reconstitute the nuggets by soaking in water. It is intended for use as training treats, snacks or as a topper for dog food.

Most of these dog food producers use fresh raw meat in their process and it comes in all the usual meats like chicken, beef, turkey, and salmon as well as more adventurous offerings like rabbit, duck, venison, and goose.

Dried dog food can be purchased from your usual pet suppliers like Petsmart or on-line through Chewy.com, Amazon.com, and similar sites. A 10 ounce bag seems to be most common and sells for $30.00 to $40.00 at the time of this writing. A 7 pound bag goes for around $85.00. Each 7 pound bag typically makes around 40 pounds of food after hydration. Use these prices for comparison only.

The DogFoodAdvisor.com web site lists over a dozen brands of dehydrated or freeze-dried dog foods. Two thirds of these brands earn 4 to 5 stars (out of 5 possible) for nutritional content. So it is possible to get a nutritionally complete freeze-dried dog food that combines meat, grain, and vegetables

Be aware, however, that recently dogs have been dying of heart disease caused by diets too high in protein. If you feed your dog almost exclusively on meat (dried or otherwise) they can develop an enlarged heart that will fail. There has been lots of discussion among veterinarians on what elements and vitamins are missing from all-meat diets. Taurine is a prime candidate (see page 96 for more on this).

Chapter 5: Raw Meat Diets

Let's face it: our domesticated canines are NOT wolves, so feeding them the diet of a wild hunter is not likely to be as beneficial as you may think. However, proponents of the raw diet do hold out benefits of a properly handled raw diet. Kimberly Morris Gauthier, author of **A Novice's Guide to Raw Feeding for Dogs** touts these benefits:

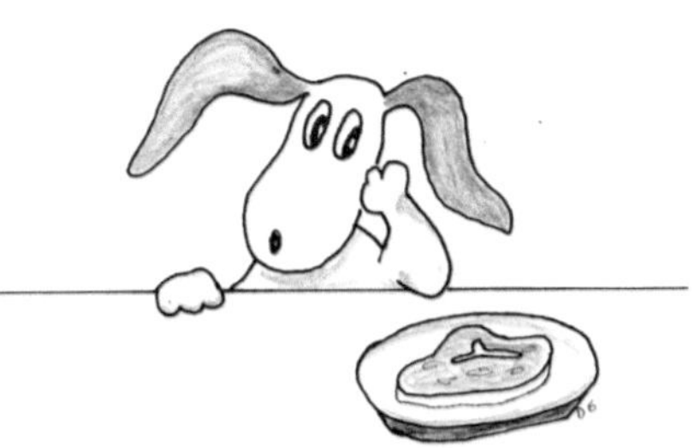

- No More Allergies – A raw food diet boosts immune system health, helping dogs combat allergies.
- Gorgeous Coat – The healthy fatty acids and nutrients in a raw diet for dogs improve their skin and coat health.
- Cleaner Teeth – Enjoying raw meaty bones satisfies the chew drive while cleaning teeth and freshening breath.
- Healthy Weight – Raw fed dogs eat natural, unprocessed foods and have more energy and focus.
- Smaller Poop – A raw diet is easier to digest, dogs absorb more nutrients, leading to smaller poop.
- Fewer Vet Visits – Switching to raw reduced vet visits from every other month to annual check-ups.

Precautions to use with any raw meat, but especially fish, will be to buy only what you can use quickly unless you freeze it. Bacterial infection grows rapidly in raw meats, so be sure your dog consumes all of the meal (or discard the remainder safely), then wash the dish in soapy water. Also be aware that meat alone does not contain all the vitamins and minerals dogs require. Wild carnivores do eat vegetation too.

Let's Start With Fish

Fish meat contains a variety of beneficial oils and nutrients, but fish are known to be infested with parasites that can transfer into your dog's muscle tissue if fed raw. To avoid this you can freeze the fish for at least a week to kill the parasites before feeding the thawed raw fish to your dog, or you can buy fish from specialty outlets such as:

- Raw Paws Pet Food - https://www.rawpawspetfood.com
- Vital Essentials Raw - http://www.vitalessentialsraw.com/
- OC Raw Dog - http://www.ocrawdog.com/

Users on discussion boards recommend against grinding raw fish because the smell hangs in the air forever. Better to dice the meat into small chunks and use it that way.

Other Meats

Typically, 5% to 8% of a raw meat diet (other than fish) should be made up of ground raw bone in order to provide an adequate amount of calcium and zinc. If you have access to a good butcher shop, they can do this for you. Otherwise you will need to buy a grinder for this.

You can utilize the muscle meat from most any animal from duck to buffalo. Common meats such as chicken, beef, and pork can be bought at your grocery store. More exotic offerings will come from suppliers or hunter friends.

Raw Feeding Models

There are several methods or “models” that are popular in raw diet feeding.

BARF Model

BARF (Biologically Appropriate Raw Food) Model Raw Feeding is a raw food diet that includes fruits, vegetables, and supplements. This is where many raw feeders start because it's easy to incorporate and many pre-made raw brands are based on the BARF model of raw feeding. BARF Model raw feeders believe that fruits and vegetables are an important part of a dog's diet and provide many nutrients that are beneficial to our dogs' health. 65%-75% muscle meat, 10%-15% bone, 5% offal, 5% liver, 5%-10% vegetables, dairy, eggs

Prey Model

Prey Model Raw Feeding is a raw food diet that includes meat, organ meat, and bone. It is claimed this model more closely resembles what wolves eat in the wild. Prey Model raw feeders believe that vegetables and fruit aren't necessary for a dog's diet and only serve as fillers. Prey Model ratio: 80% muscle meat, 10% bone, 5% offal, 5% liver.

FrankenBARF Model

This is mostly BARF Model with some Prey Model mixed in. Many raw feeders have found that vegetables and fruit are a beneficial part of their dogs' diet. Some also add supplements to their meals. The FrankenBARF Model ratio is 80% muscle meat, 10% bone, 5% offal, 5% liver. Vegetables, goats milk, raw eggs, supplements – all added in to the above to provide additional nutrients and satisfy each dog's specific needs.

Commercial Premade Raw

Premade raw dog food refers to commercially prepared raw dog food. The benefit of feeding premade raw is that it reduces the concern about sourcing and feeding a balanced diet – the brand takes care of this for you. However, because the brand takes on the burden of providing a quality, balanced raw diet – they charge a premium price for their food. There are a lot of new brands coming to the market that practice questionable sourcing, use synthetic vitamins, and aren't transparent about their ingredients. Beware of these, do your homework. Trusted brands include Darwin's Natural Pet Products, Answers Pet Food, Columbia Pet Food, Raw Paws Pet Food, and GreenTripe.com.

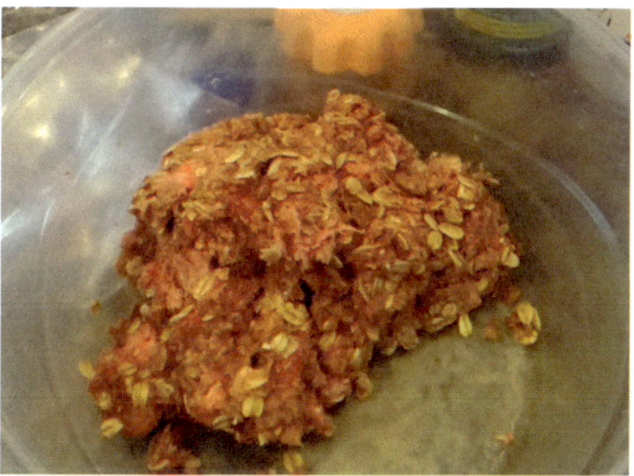

NOTES:

Chapter 6: Making Bone Broth

Bone broth has many health benefits. Bone broth has been traditionally used to treat leaky gut and digestive issues, while also supporting good joint health. It benefits dogs with allergies and food sensitivities, as it is an immune system booster. For healthy dogs, a ladle of bone broth over kibble once a day is an excellent whole food multivitamin.

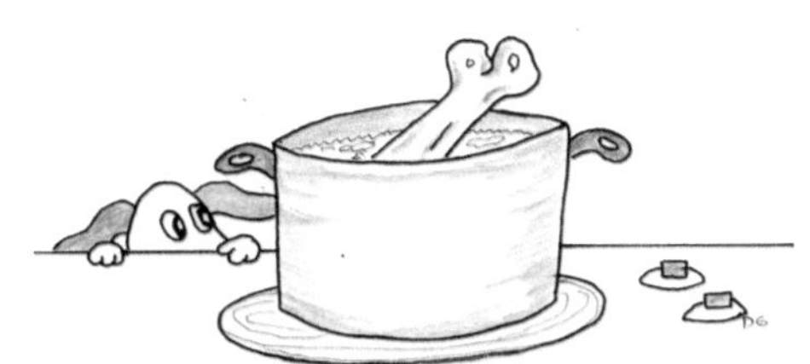

Bone broth is rich in many nutrients, especially amino acids such as arginine, glycine, glutamine and proline. Bone broth also acts as a superior joint supplement, as it contains gelatin (the breakdown of collagen), glucosamine, and chondroitin that support good joint health.

Protein rich bone broth contains vitamin C, vitamin D, vitamin K, iron, thiamin, potassium, calcium, silicon, sulfer, magnesium, glucosamine, phosphorus, trace minerals, and glucosamine chondroitin sulfates.

It's easy to make too – even if you don't normally cook. If you have a crock pot you can make bone broth. Basically you just simmer meat bones in water for 8 to 24 hours. If you can boil water you can make bone broth.

1) Start with a large crock pot or a stock pot. Put in this around two pounds of bones. You can use any kind of bones: raw or cooked, poultry, beef, or pork: they all work fine, but joint bones work better than straight leg bone segments.

If you are using something like beef marrow bones (disks cut from cow leg bones) that have little or no cartilage to them, add a few chicken feet. If you're using a turkey carcass, that has plenty of cartilage to provide the glucosamine and condroitan.

2) Cover the bones with enough water to be 3" above the top of the bones.

3) Add 3 or 4 tablespoons of either apple cider vinegar or lemon juice. This acidifies the water to help pull the best nutrients out of the bones.

4) Cover and heat on high until the water comes to a rolling boil. NOTE: your crock pot may not be capable of this. Not to worry, just extend the cooking time.

5) Reduce heat to maintain a simmer and keep covered. How long you cook it depends on whether you're using a crock pot or stock pot and what kind of bones you're using. Heavy bones will need to cook longer than a turkey carcass. A crock pot will need to cook overnight because of the lower temperature is uses. A turkey

carcass in a stock pot, brought to boiling then reduced should finish up in around 8 hours.

6) When the cooking time is completed, let the stock cool a bit before going to the next step.

7) Strain the bones and meat out of the stock either by fishing them out with a slotted spoon or by pouring the stock through a strainer or colander into a large bowl or another pot. Put the container of stock in your refrigerator to chill.

8) Discard the bones. Even if they are beef or pork bones, do not give them to your dog no matter how much she pleads. All the "good" has been cooked out of them now and having been weakened they won't be much good as a chew bone.

9) OPTIONAL: go through the stuff in your strainer and fish out the bits of meat. Discard solid bones (chicken and turkey bones come out soft and friable, you can safely crush these into the meat), skin and globs of fat (these are bad fat and promote pancreatitis in dogs). Cartilage is okay if you want to keep it: it adds texture that some dogs like. This "good stuff" can be put back into the completed broth or stored separately and used in your dog food recipes (see chapter 7).

10) Once your broth has chilled, take it out of the fridge. It will have a hard layer of fat on top. Chip that off and discard it (see note about fat and pancreatitis in step 9 above).

Underneath the fat your bone broth should now look like jelly. The stiff consistency means you've got lots of gelatin in there and that's what helps keep your dog's joints moving well. That gelatin plugs the holes in a leaky gut that can cause allergy symptoms, so the more jelly-like, the better!

If your broth doesn't look like jelly, it just means you didn't add enough vinegar. Next time add a little more vinegar and that batch should be just fine.

Depending on how much broth you made and how much you will use (how many dogs you have and what size) you may need to put some of the chilled broth in a zipper bag and freeze it. This won't keep long, so don't keep more than a few days worth in the fridge.

This bone broth can be used as "gravy" on top of kibble (Chapter 2), or as an ingredient of doggie stew (Chapter 3), over a raw diet (Chapter 5), or in a bowl as a stand-alone meal as long as it's part of a balanced diet plan.

Chapter 7: Home-Cooked Recipes

In this chapter I'll present a series of recipes that can serve as a launching point for your own experimentation. If you've read the previous chapters on nutrition, you should have a good handle on how to keep things in line. Remember that every meal does not have to be "formula perfect" in regards to nutritional content. Take a "big picture" approach and shoot for a balanced diet over time.

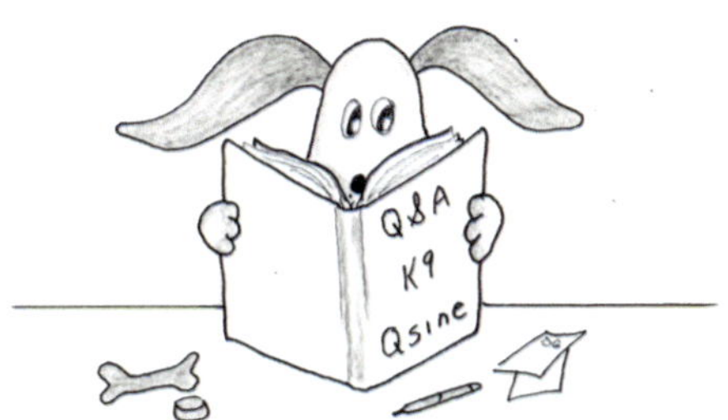

Use the recipes included here as templates into which you can plug-in different meats, green veggies, starches, and good grains.

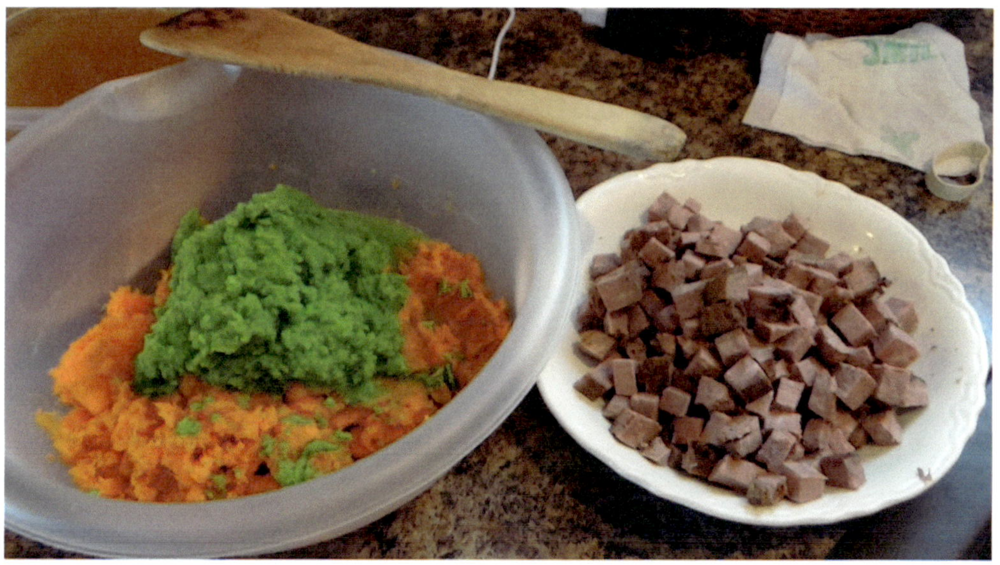

Doing the Math on Servings

What happens when a recipe is calculated for a 50 pound dog and you have a 38 pound dog? Or a 79 pound dog? How do you adjust your servings? You can always fall back on the general rule of thumb of 2% to 3% of your dogs body weight, then measure the food out on a kitchen scale. Or you can divide out the recipe recommendation on an ounces per pound basis.

WARNING: *I'm rounding things off here because, let's face it: working with food is not like precise chemical formulas where one drop too much of methyl-floride-acetate will blow you and your whole lab sky high. Yes, I made that name up: I'm no chemist. The point is we don't need to get into advanced mathematics to cook.*

In the following Ground Beef and Broccoli recipe the daily serving of just under 3 cups (it's actually 2 5/6 cups + 1 Tbs, which is 1/16 of a cup) is for a 50 pound dog. But we don't want to work in fractions of a cup, so let's use fluid ounces.

- There are 8 fl. oz. in one cup.
- 8 oz. per cup x 3 cups (see above) of food = 24 fl. oz. of food per serving.
- The daily serving for a 50 pound dog is 24 fluid ounces (using a measuring cup not a scale). If we divide 24 ounces of food by the 50 pounds of dog we get just a smidge under ½ ounce per pound.
- If your dog is 38 pounds, using the ½ fl. oz./ lb formula, you can multiply 38 pounds by ½ (0.5 in calculator speak) fluid ounces and get 19 fluid ounces which is 2 1/3 cups.
- A 79 pound dog would get 79 x 0.5 = 39.5 oz. divided by 8 ounces per cup = 4.94 cups. Call it 5 cups per daily serving.

Easy right?

Or you can buy a good kitchen scale and weigh the food out in pounds and ounces. That's what I do. Fewer headaches that way.

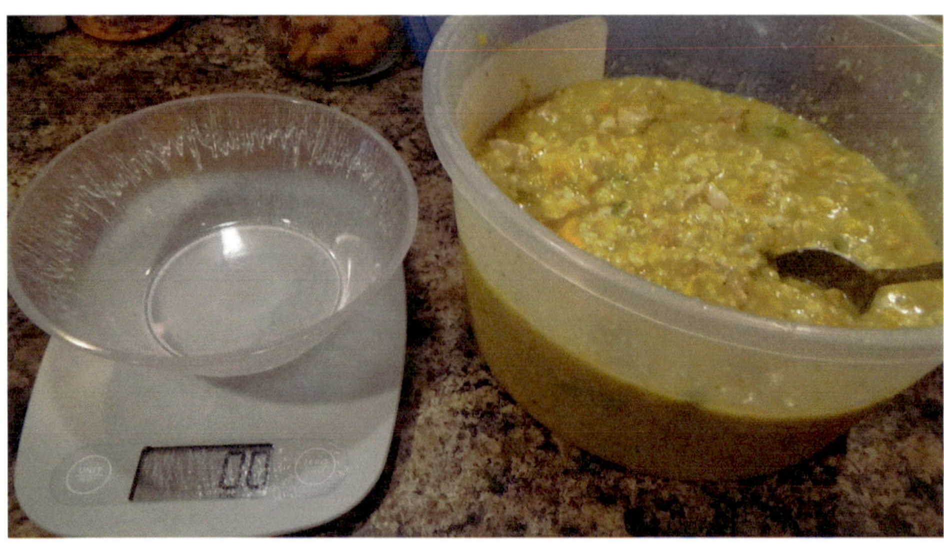

Ground Beef and Broccoli

When wading into an unfamiliar process it's best to start with something simple, so here's a delightfully simple recipe that will make 4 servings for a 50 pound dog.

Ingredients:

2 pounds lean ground beef
1 cup broccoli florets (chopped)
1 cup uncooked oatmeal
1 tablespoon olive oil
2000 mg calcium citrate

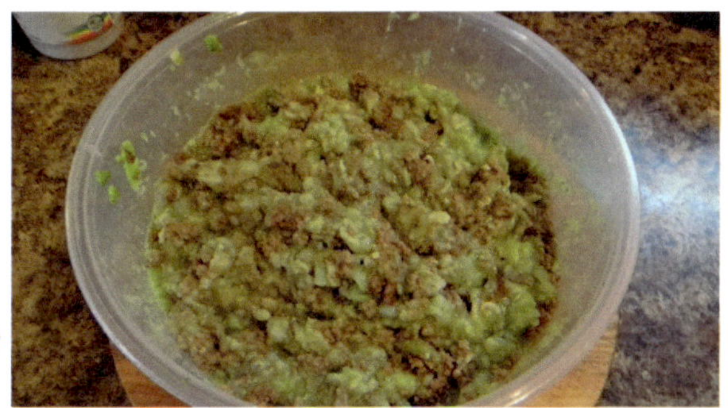

Note: If you are using beef ground for dogs (with bones ground in) omit the additional calcium.

Directions

Heat the oil in a large skillet over medium-low heat. Add the ground beef and cook until it is browned. Drain the fat, mix the calcium into the meat as it cools.

Prepare the oatmeal according to package directions. When cooked it should produce about 2 cups. Set it aside to cool.

Steam the broccoli until semi-tender then finely chop it in a blender or food processor. You should end up with ¼ cup of broccoli.

Serving

At this point you have the option of storing each ingredient in a separate container and mixing them up when you serve it to your dog (for a 50 pound dog: 1 1/3 cup beef, ½ cup oatmeal, 1 Tbs broccoli for one daily serving. If you feed twice a day, split this.) or you can mix it all together now and put it in one container (kept in the fridge) and serve your dog just shy of 3 cups per day, or divide it up equally into 4 containers and store them in the fridge until used.

These portions are for a 50 pound dog. If you have a 25 pound dog, you will get 8 portions of 1½ cups each.

NOTES:

Broccoli Beef Sweet Potato Doggie Stew

Ingredients

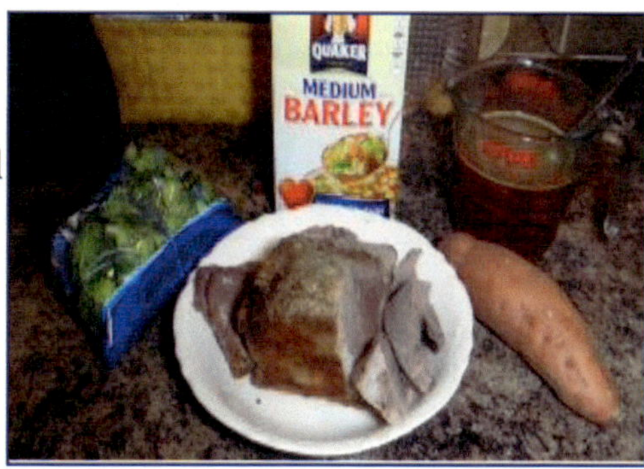

- 2 cups cooked beef cut into 1/4" cubes
- 1½ cups of chopped broccoli
- 2 or 3 large sweet potato (needs to yield 2 cups when mashed)
- ½ cup uncooked barley
- 4 cups liquid (including beef broth)
- 1000 mg calcium citrate

Directions

Steam the veggies until soft. Don't boil them. Then mash or puree to release the nutrients, a dog's gut does not break down cellulose like ours do, so they can't get at the nutrients of many plants, especially leafy plants. Use some water for thinning the puree so it renders down smoothly. Chopping it finely in a food processor also works well.

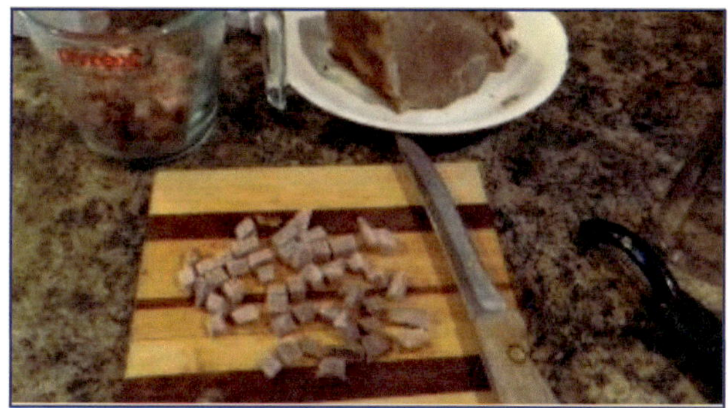

Cube up your beef. Cut it into small pieces that won't choke your dog (they are not known for chewing their food well) and will be easily digested. Trim away excess fat. Large amounts of meat fat causes pancreatitis in dogs.

Boil up the barley according to package directions. You may have to do some math here -- or just make a larger amount and save the excess in the fridge for the next batch. Use some beef broth to cook the barley. If you need to drain off excess liquid after cooking, use a strainer and bowl to capture the liquid, don't pour it down the drain. That has good stuff in it, don't waste it. You need two cups of cooked barley. Mash it well, use broth to thin as needed. Add the mashed sweet potatoes.

Add the calcium citrate. If you have the gel-caps, pull them apart and add the powder. If a tablet, crush them in a pull crusher or between two large, nested spoons. Calcium is important to your dog's diet. A wild dog gets calcium by eating the bones of its prey. We need to add calcium citrate or (dietary) bone meal to the recipes. Mix it through well.

Add meat cubes and the chopped or pureed broccoli. Mix but don’t blend.

Go ahead and give it a taste, everything you've used is human grade food so just because you're calling it dog food doesn't mean you can't try a bit. I can definitely taste the sweet potato, the broccoli is more subtle.

Okay, pack that into an air-tight container and store it in the fridge. If you have any liquid left, save that too, you'll need it for thinning in days to come: it will stiffen up as it sits.

Pork Necks and Green Beans

This recipe was given to me by my friend Macey Fortney. Her dogs Monster and Chloe love it.

Ingredients

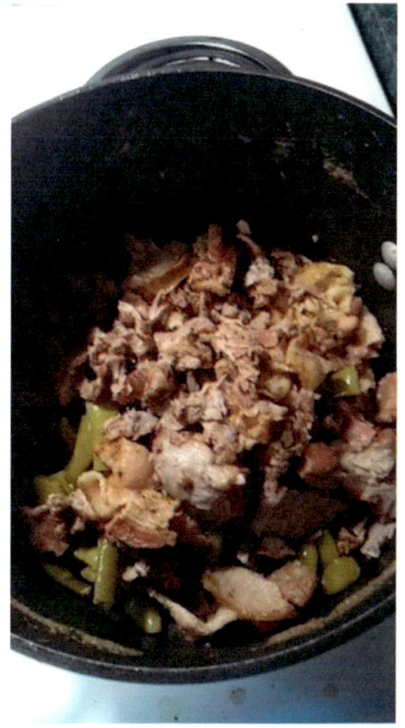

- Package of pork necks
- Bacon
- Frozen green beans
- Rice
- Flour or cornstarch

Directions

Boil the pork necks all day and pull the meat off. Save the liquid.

Cook up the bacon, drain the grease off into your bacon grease jar. You DO have a bacon grease jar, right? You can't be a true Southerner without a bacon grease jar. When cool, crumble the bacon.

Steam the green beans until tender and chop them up. Toss them in a little hot bacon grease (see, I told you you were going to need that grease) for a few seconds just to flavor them..

Boil up the rice according to package directions. Then mash it into mush.

Make a rue from flour or cornstarch and make gravy from some of the pork neck fluid.

Mix gravy into the rice, keeping it nice and loose, add green beans, bacon crumbles, and top with pork meat.

YUM!

NOTES:

Skinny Dog Stew

Chicken fat is an excellent source of fatty acids as well as caloric content. This recipe is made for fattening up a scrawny or emaciated dog. If your dog is at a healthy weight, eliminate the chicken fat.

Ingredients

- 1 chicken
- 4 cups of chopped spinach
- 4 medium potatoes (needs to yield 3 cups when mashed)
- 1½ cups uncooked oats
- 3 cups water
- 2 Tbsp flax seed oil
- 1,500 mg calcium citrate

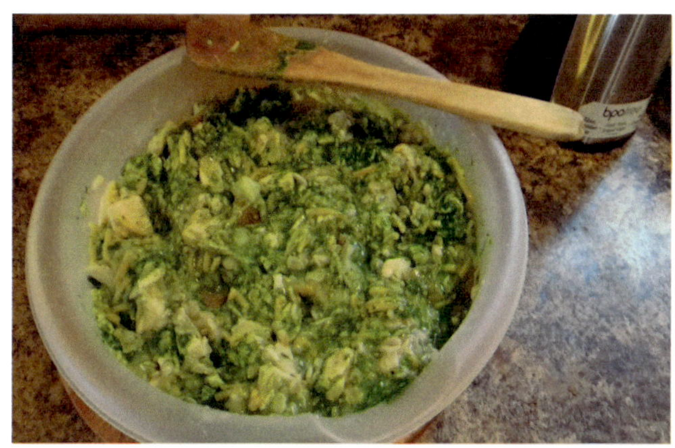

Directions

Roast or boil your chicken. Let cool enough to handle and remove meat from the bones and shred or chop it. Add the Calcium Citrate powder to 3 cups of the meat. Freeze remaining meat for use another time.

Discard the chicken skin. Let the broth sit in the fridge so the fat rises and gels. Skim that off and mix it back into the meat. Reserve the liquid for use. Refrigerate or freeze the bones for making bone broth.

Scrub the potatoes well. Remove any bad spots but leave the skins on. Poke the skins with a fork and microwave the potatoes until soft (3 runs of 3 minutes each, turning the spuds over after each run does it in my microwave. Yours may vary.), cut into chunks and mash them. Yes, skins and all, a lot of a potatoes nutrients are right under the skin.

Steam the spinach until tender. Don't boil it. Then chop or puree to release the nutrients, a dog's gut does not break down cellulose like ours do, so they can't get at the nutrients of leafy plants. Use some of the broth for thinning the puree so it renders down smoothly. Chopping can be done without added liquid.

Boil up the oats according to package directions. You want them kind of loose (runny) not stiff. Then puree them to make them digestible for dogs.

With the mashed potatoes in a large bowl, add the oat mush and mix well. Add the chicken, add the spinach and stir just enough to mix. It does not need to be blended into a homogeneous monotone mass. Thin with chicken stock as you mix to give it a slightly soupy texture. If you roasted the chicken and run out of broth, thin with water.

Pack that into an air-tight container and store it in the fridge. If you have any chicken broth left, save that too, you'll need it for thinning in days to come: it will stiffen up as it sits.

Satin Balls

A raw meat recipe by shangrilarcadia on Instructibles.com

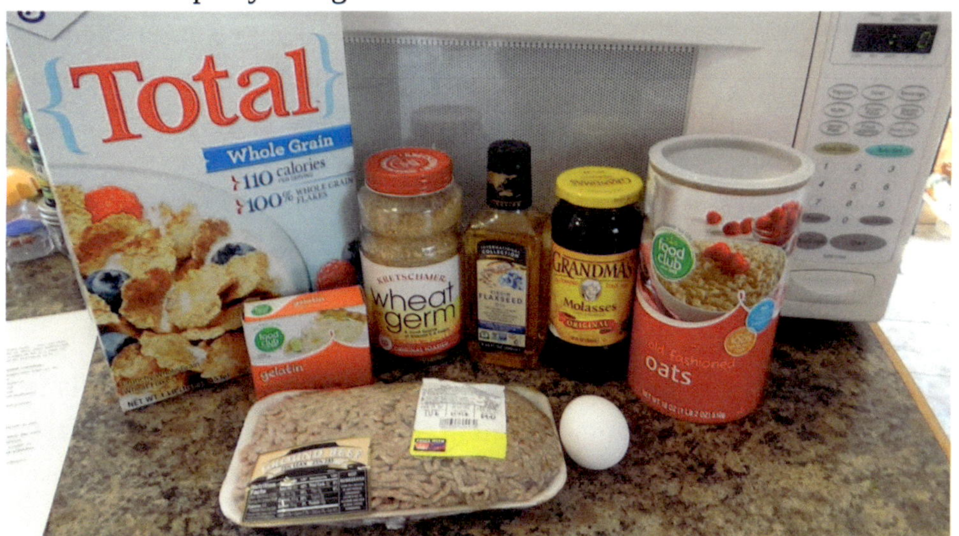

One of the best ways to put weight on a dog is with something called "satin balls". You can find the recipe on many web sites on the internet. Some people use it to put weight on their dogs before dog shows, but it's especially good for emaciated dogs and dogs who won't eat. It's high in fat so it puts on weight quickly, but it's also got other ingredients to make it a total diet so it can be fed alone or as a supplement.

This is the original version:

- 10 pounds hamburger (the cheapest kind)
- 1 lg. box of Total cereal
- 1 lg. box oatmeal
- 1 jar of wheat germ
- 1 1/4 cup Flax oil
- 1 1/4 cup of unsulphured molasses
- 10 raw eggs AND shells
- 10 envelopes of unflavored gelatin
- pinch of salt

This is a scaled down trial version:

- 1 pound cheap hamburger (for high fat %)
- 1 1/3 cups Total cereal
- 1 1/2 cups uncooked oatmeal
- 6 tablespoons wheat germ
- 2 tablespoons flax seed oil
- 2 tablespoons unsulphured molasses
- 1 raw egg
- 1 envelope Knox unflavored gelatin
- pinch of salt

Directions

Note on the egg: The shell is to be included for its calcium, but to avoid cutting the throat or gut, crush the shell well. Calcium Carbonate (egg shell) is more concentrated but not as readily absorbed by a dog as Calcium Citrate. Personally, I save the shells for my garden and feed the dogs Calcium Citrate.

Mix everything together in a big bowl. I recommend putting the dry ingredients first, then the oils, then the egg, then the meat. That way you don't have to wash your hands in between ingredients.

You can form this into balls like the name suggests, but I prefer patties because they are easier to stack in the freezer. How much you put into each serving depends on the size of your dog and whether these are to be treats or meals. For my emaciated Greyhound (target weight 50 pounds) I used ½ pound satin balls fed with a half-portion of stew in the evening (straight Skinny Dog Stew for breakfast and lunch) and her hips, shoulder blades, and ribs disappeared under healthy flesh quickly.

Lay the patties in bags and freeze them. Since they are served raw you need to thaw individually when you are ready to serve them. Bag accordingly.

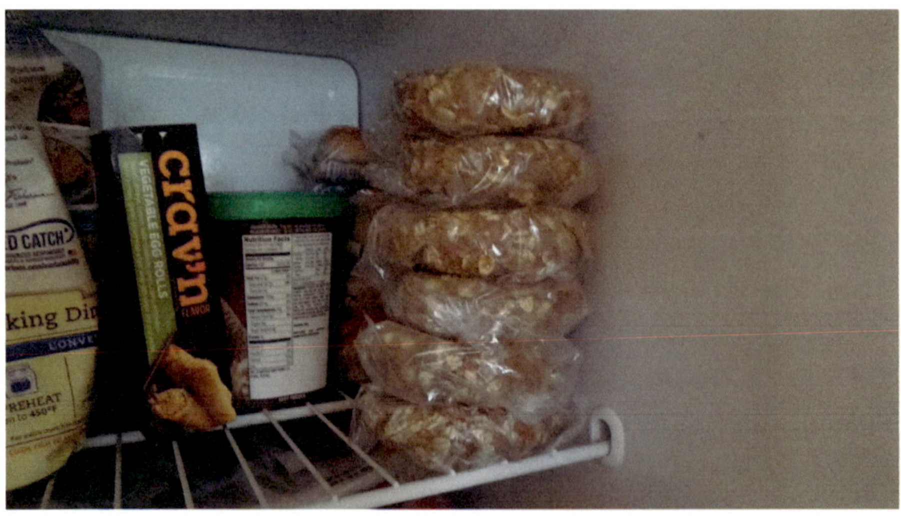

Chicken, Cheese, and Squash Stew

Ingredients

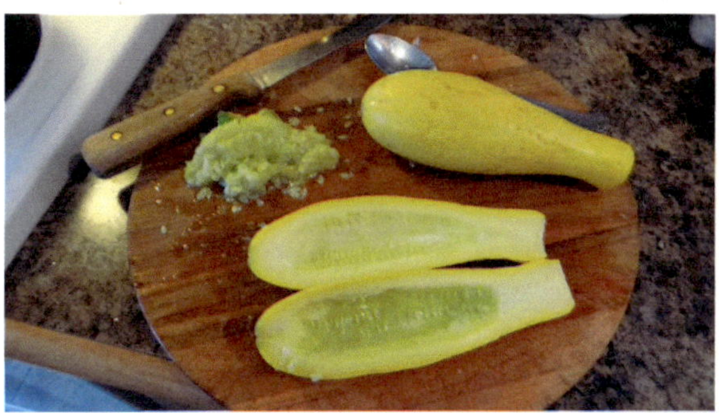

- 2 cups boiled and diced chicken (about 2 pounds raw chicken breast, a little more with bones)
- 1 cup low fat cheddar cheese
- 2½ cups raw broccoli (will cook down to 2 cups)
- 2 cups cooked and mashed squash
- 1¼ cup uncooked brown rice
- 10 cups water
- 2 Tbs Flax seed oil
- 2000 mg Calcium Citrate

Directions

Follow the package directions to cook 3 cups of rice. Usually this is 1 cup of rice to 2 cups of water and cook for 45-50 minutes.

Boil the chicken in the remaining water. Chicken breasts generally take 20 to 25 minutes to cook through.

Remove the chicken from the water (now broth) and reserve the liquid. Allow the chicken pieces to drain and cool enough to handle, then dice or shred the meat. Preserve the bones for making bone broth. If you end up with more than the two cups of meat, label and freeze the remainder for use later, or if it's a small amount, just feed it to the dogs who are no doubt gathered around watching you. There is no point in torturing them!

Add the Calcium Citrate and mix through the meat.

Steam or microwave the broccoli, then finely chop or puree.

Half, seed, and roast or microwave the squash. Scoop flesh from the rind. Measure out the 2 cups you need, store the remainder.

In a large bowl combine rice, squash, and flax oil. Use broth to thin as needed.

Stir in chicken and cheese.

Stir in broccoli.

Place a measuring cup on your kitchen scale and zero the scale. Spoon stew into the measuring cup until the scale reads 1 pound. Record the level in the measuring cup. Use this measurement in calculating portions based on your dog's weight, as described earlier.

Place in air tight containers and refrigerate.

NOTES:

Pork, Peas and Quinoa

This one uses peas as a bridge between vegetables and protein because they are both. You can substitute chick peas or legumes for the peas to change things up without disrupting the recipe.

Ingredients

- 1½ lbs raw pork
- 1 cup uncooked quinoa
- 2 cups fresh or frozen peas
- 3 medium sweet potatoes
- 1,500 mg Calcium Citrate
- 2 Tbsp Flax seed oil
- Water

Directions

If your peas are frozen, place the sealed package in a bowl of cool water to thaw.

Remove any excess fat from the pork and cook the meat. Depending on the cut you're using you can boil it (save the broth) or roast it in the oven or a crock pot, or if you're really talented, you can cook it in the microwave. While it's cooking prepare your other ingredients.

Put the quinoa in a colander and rinse well under cold water to remove the bitter coating (unless you bought pre-rinsed quinoa - it will say on the package). Drain well and place the clean grain in a medium sauce pan. Add 2¼ cups of water and put on the stove at medium-high heat until it starts to boil. When it boils, reduce heat to low, cover the pan, and cook for 12-15 minutes. Remove from heat. I like to let it sit a while to make sure it absorbs all the liquid it will. There should be a little water left. That's to help as you mash that lovely quinoa into paste (groan). The doggoes guts have a hard time with whole grains so we have to mash it well to make sure it's digestible for them.

Cook the sweet potatoes until soft. Again, you can roast them in the oven or microwave them. I find three rounds of 4 minutes each, turning them between rounds, does a nice job in the microwave. When done, split in half let them cool until workable and scoop the 'tater out of the skin. Measure out 3 cups to use, refrigerate or freeze the rest for use another time.

Steam the two cups of peas until soft, then puree.

Dice or shred the pork. Mix the calcium citrate through the meat. Use 2 cups of meat, preserve any remainder.

In a large bowl combine the quinoa and sweet potato. Use the pork broth (or water) to thin as needed to get a soupy stew consistency. Add the flax seed oil and stir through. Add the pork and mix in. Thin it a little more if needed. Finally add the pureed peas and stir them in. It looks nicer if you leave it a little colorful, not a homogenized shade. The dogs don't care, but where's the artistry in that?

Place in a sealed container and store in the refrigerator. Keep any remaining broth for thinning again tomorrow.

Another Raw Meat Recipe

This one was developed by Dr. Karen Becker and Rodney Habib.

Ingredients

- 14 oz raw ground beef that is at least 90% lean (for high amino acid value)
- 1 oz raw beef liver (copper, iron, zinc)
- ½ can (2 oz) sardines packed in water, no salt added
- 2 tsp Hemp seed oil (to balance fats in the meat)
- ½ tsp Kelp powder (for iodine)
- ½ tsp Ginger powder (manganese)
- 1 oz fresh Broccoli
- 1 oz Red bell pepper
- 1 oz raw Spinach
- 1 raw egg (wash the shell first)

Directions

Place the raw ground beef and egg in a bowl. Add hemp seed oil, kelp, and ginger.

In a food processor, place sardines, ½ egg shell, beef liver, broccoli, bell pepper, and spinach. Pulse until blended. Then add to contents of the bowl and stir thoroughly.

Feeding

Portion this out using the 2% to 3% of body weight per day feeding schedule. This is designed for an adult dog, a puppy would need more calcium. Keep no more than 2 days worth of this food in the fridge, freeze the rest. I'd recommend freezing individual portions in zip-lock bags.

Please note: This is not a balanced recipe. Being heavy on protein, if made into a steady diet you could send your dog into heart failure. I include it as published as a "change of pace" recipe. Once in a while will be fine, but I don't recommend making a habit of feeding this style of dog food.

NOTES:

Ground Beef, Mashed Potatoes, and Broccoli

Just good home cooking for your furry friends

Ingredients:

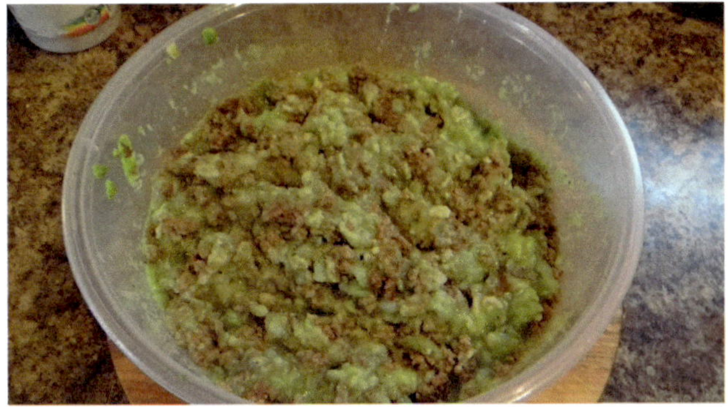

- 1¾ lbs lean ground beef
- 2½ Cups chopped and tightly packed fresh broccoli (may include stems)
- 3 Medium baking potatoes
- 1½ Cups uncooked oats
- 2 Tbsp Flax seed oil
- 2,000 mg Calcium Citrate
- Approximately 5 cups of water

Directions

Place 2½ cups of water in a large sauce pan and bring to a boil. Add 1½ cups of raw oats, reduce heat and cook, uncovered, for 5 minutes. Remove from heat, cover and let sit for a few minutes.

Scrub your potatoes. Poke the potatoes with a fork and place them in the microwave on high for 3 minutes. Turn them over and microwave for another 3 minutes. Repeat until soft (usually 3 rounds does it for me). Allow to cool until you can handle them, then dice (skins and all) and put in a large bowl.

Add the oats and mash both well. This should be rather soupy. If it's too stiff, add more water.

Add 2 Tbsp Flax seed oil and mix through.

Place chopped broccoli in a glass bowl with ¼ cup water. Cover and microwave for 3-4 minutes to steam the broccoli. Place softened broccoli and ¼ cup water in a blender or food processor and puree. Add puree to the mixture in the large bowl.

Brown the ground beef in a pan and drain off and discard the grease. Mix the Calcium Citrate through the meat. Add the meat to the bowl and mix. Add water to thin if needed.

Pack the stew into air tight containers and store in the fridge. This will make about a gallon of stew. If you have a small dog, keep out enough for 3 days, package the rest into containers or freezer bags - each with about 3 days worth in them – and freeze. Bring them back out as you need them. At Piney Mountain Foster Care, a gallon of stew lasts two days, so I just keep it in one large container in the fridge.

NOTES:

Beef Bonanza

A crock-pot recipe by Amy downs of www.topdogtips.com

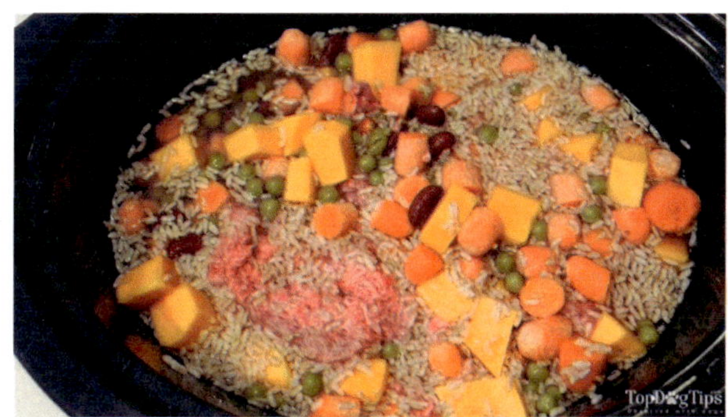

Prep Time: 10 minutes
Cook Time: 6 hours

Ingredients:

- 2½ pounds of lean ground beef
- 1½ cup of brown rice
- 1 15-ounce can of kidney beans, drained and rinsed
- 1½ cup of chopped butternut squash
- 1½ cup of chopped carrots
- ½ cup of frozen or canned peas

Directions

Combine all ingredients in the crock pot and add four cups of water. Once everything is well mixed, cover the crock pot and cook the meal at low heat for about 6 hours. Alternatively, you can cook at high heat for 2 or 3 hours, but you'll need to stir regularly.

Once the stew is ready, let it cool off completely. Then, it will be ready to serve or package and be put in the freezer.

Side note: If you are concerned about the fat content of ground beef, replace it with diced chicken or ground turkey.

NOTES:

Beef and Pork Crock Pot Dog Food

By Samantha Randall of www.topdogtips.com

Ingredients

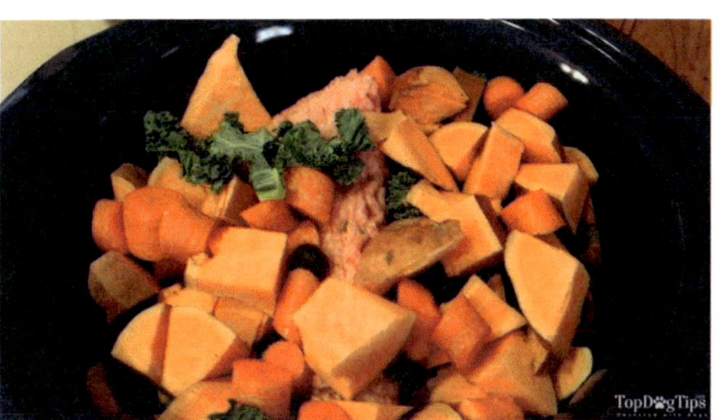

- 1.5 cups water
- 1 cup brown rice
- 4 lbs. protein source (I used 1 lb. ground beef and 3 lbs. ground pork)
- 1/2 cup blueberries
- 1 large apple (cubed)
- 1 cup kale (chopped)
- 1 large sweet potato (cubed)
- 2 large carrots (cut into chunks)

Directions

As with most slow cooker recipes, this one is very simple to make. It takes me about 15 minutes to cut up all the fruits and vegetables for this recipe, and that's all the work you need to do.

Just add all the ingredients to your slow cooker and stir the dog food occasionally as it cooks. You can cook this recipe for 4 hours on the 'high' setting or 7 hours on the 'low' setting.

I usually use frozen meat in my crock pot recipes. It saves me the time of defrosting the meat, and it won't change the taste or texture of the food at all. Just add about 30-45 minutes to your cook time if you use frozen meat.

NOTES:

Doggie Stew

A crockpot recipe by Amy Downs of www.topdogtips.com

Prep time: 15 minutes
Cook time: 6 to 12 hours

Ingredients:

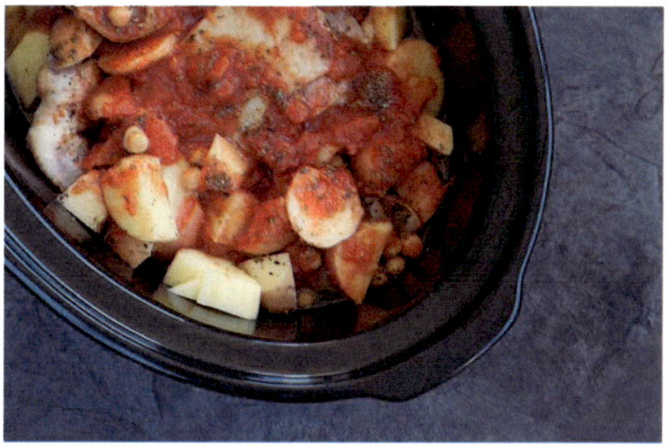

- 3 pounds of boneless and skinless chicken thighs (this roughly equals 10 to 12 medium-sized thighs)
- ¼ cup of cup chicken livers
- 2 peeled and sliced medium-sized carrots
- 1 cup of frozen green beans
- 1 big apple or 2 medium-sized apples (remove the core and seeds and cut the apples into pieces)
- 2 to 3 cups of water
- 1 cup of frozen peas
- 1 handful of chopped, fresh parsley
- 1 tablespoon of olive oil

Directions:

Put the chicken thighs into the slow cooker. Add chicken livers, carrots, beans, apples, and water to it. The water needs to be just enough to cover the rest of the ingredients and not more. Cover the pot and cook on low heat for 8 hours (or on higher heat for 2-3 hours, but you'll need to stir frequently; this depends on your slow cooker, too).

10 – 15 minutes before the meal is cooked, add the peas, parsley and olive oil. Once everything is cooked, let it cool off completely. After that, it's ready to serve or be put in the freezer.

Side note: Remember that while apples are good for dogs, apple seeds are toxic, so it is crucial to remove the core and the seeds from the apple(s). This generally applies to all fruits and vegetables. Also, to prevent choking with any of these homemade crockpot dog food recipes, you are strongly advised to remove the bones from the thighs (or to use deboned chicken).

Veggie Protein Blast

A crockpot recipe by Amy Downs of www.topdogtips.com

Prep time: 15 minutes
Cook time: 12 hours

Ingredients:

- 3 pounds of chicken thighs
- 3 pounds of ground turkey
- 2 small, diced potatoes
- 2 small, diced sweet potatoes
- 8 ounces of frozen peas
- 8 ounces of chopped carrots
- 1 cup of frozen blueberries

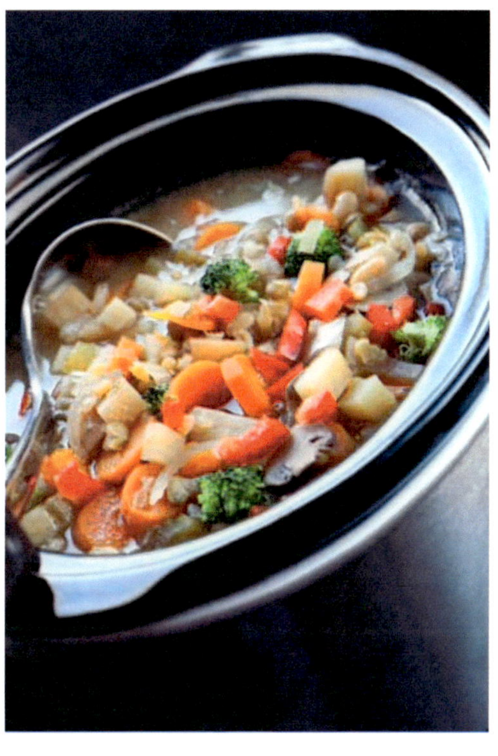

Directions:

The ground turkey and the chicken thighs are to be placed first in the crockpot. Pour just enough water to cover them completely. After that, add the rest of the ingredients and cover the slow cooker. Cook your slow cooker dog food meal like this on a low heat for 12 hours. I do not recommended to cook on a higher heat because it will require constant stirring and it will still take several hours.

Once the crock pot dog food meal is ready, let it cool off. Remove the bones from the chicken in order to prevent choking. Once that's done, the dish is ready to be served or to be frozen in portions for later use. Once again, remember that if you're not using any commercial dog foods then ask your veterinarian about this specific recipe and any supplements you must add to suit your dog's health conditions.

NOTES:

Acorn Squash, Chicken, and Barley

A light meal your dog will love

Ingredients

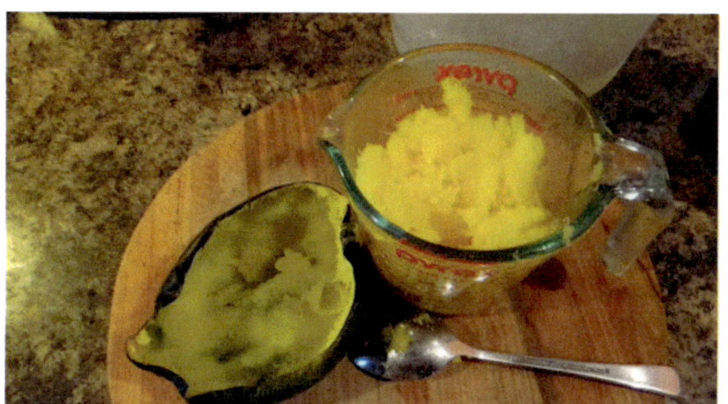

- 1 large Acorn Squash
- 4 cups chicken broth
- 4½ cups water
- ¾ cup raw barley
- 3 cups diced, cooked, chicken breast (approx 1½ pounds raw)
- 1 broccoli stalk
- 2 Tbsp flax seed oil
- 2000 mg calcium citrate

Directions

Bring 4 cups of water to a boil in a large pan. Add barley, stir, cover, reduce heat and simmer for 50 minutes. Pour into a large bowl and mash.

Put your chicken breasts in a large pot and cover with water. Boil until cooked through. Remove breasts and cool before dicing. Reserve the broth.

Cut the acorn squash in half and remove seeds with a spoon. Place squash in microwave and cook on high for 4 minutes. Spin squash around and cook another 4 minutes. Do this 3 times. Allow to cool before handling, then remove from the microwave and scoop flesh from the rind with a large spoon and mash. You should get 3 cups of mashed squash.

Chop your stalk of broccoli and steam it until tender. I do this by putting it in a glass bowl with ½ cup water, cover with a small plate and microwave on high for 3 minutes. Put the steamed broccoli and any water remaining in a blender and finely chop or puree. You should get 1½ cup.

Mix the mashed squash into the barley in the large bowl. Thin with chicken broth as needed. Add flax seed oil, calcium citrate, and broccoli and mix well. Stir in the diced chicken.

Place in an air tight container and store in the fridge.

Save any remaining chicken broth as well, this will stiffen up as it sits and will need to be thinned again.

NOTES:

Simple Chicken Breast & Rice

A crockpot recipe by Amy Downs of www.topdogtips.com

Prep time: 15 minutes
Cook time: 5 to 8 hours

Ingredients:

- 1 cup of brown rice
- 2 cups of water
- ½ pound of green beans, broken into segments
- 1 medium-sized, raw sweet potato (cut it into chunks, but leave the skin on)
- 3 sliced carrots
- 2 deboned chicken breasts with or without skin

Directions:

Layer all the ingredients in a crockpot in the above listed order. Chicken breasts should be on top. Cover all of them with water and start cooking. On a low heat around 8 hours should be enough. With higher heat, you can cook for just 5 hours or possibly even less, but with frequent stirring. Once your slow cooker dog food meal is cooked, mix and stir the ingredients once again. Break the chicken into small pieces and make sure that everything is soft. After that, let the dish cool off completely and it will be ready to serve or to be put in the freezer for later us.

Side note: You can substitute some of the ingredients. Broccoli florets, zucchini, spinach or squash can all work quite well in this slow cooker dog food recipe. You can also swap the chicken breasts with turkey, beef, or lamb, but be careful not to increase the fat content of the dish too much. As with all homemade crock pot dog food recipes, remember to add the vitamins, minerals and calcium supplements recommended by your veterinarian if you plan on making this dish a major part of your dog's diet. Otherwise, mix with commercial dog food for a well-balanced diet.

NOTES:

Chicken, Cheese & Green Pepper

This recipe uses our basic nutritional template but gets a little more adventurous.

Ingredients

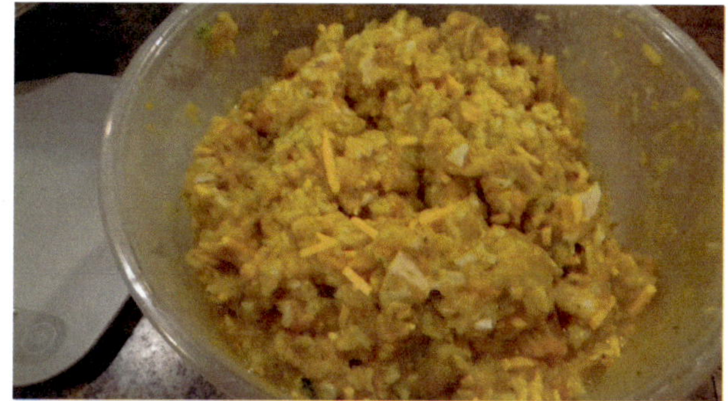

- 2 cups cooked and diced chicken breast (about 2 pounds raw meat)
- 1 cup shredded low-fat cheddar cheese
- 1 cup white rice
- 2½ cups water
- 1 medium green bell pepper
- 1 cup chopped mustard greens
- 3 medium sweet potatoes
- 2 Tbsp Flax seed oil
- 2000 mg Calcium Citrate

Directions

Poke the skins of your sweet potatoes several times and place in the microwave. Cook on high for 4 minutes, rotate and cook for another 4 minutes, repeat this until soft. (3 times usually does it for my microwave). Alternatively, you can roast them in the oven if you prefer.

While you're working on this, put the 2½ cups of water in a large sauce pan and heat to a boil. Add the rice, reduce heat to a simmer and cover. Cook according to package directions (usually 5 minutes). Leave covered and remove from heat.

Core and slice the pepper into spears. Drop the spears into your food processor to chop or puree. Don't add water this time, the pepper contains plenty. When this is done, add the mustard greens and blend together with the pepper.

Mix your Calcium Citrate through the meat.

When the potatoes are done, remove with a mitt, slice each in half lengthwise and let cool enough to handle. Then scoop the flesh out of the skins. Discard the skins. Measure out 3 cups of sweet potato. Preserve any remainder for some other use.

Pour the rice into a large bowl (it should be a little soupy) and mash it well. Add the sweet potato and mash again. Add the flax seed oil, green puree, and chicken breast. Mix well. If it's too stiff, thin with water. Add the cheese and stir it through.

Place in an airtight container and place in refrigerator.

Pork, Summer Squash and Mustard Greens

A Southern dish for your doggo

Ingredients

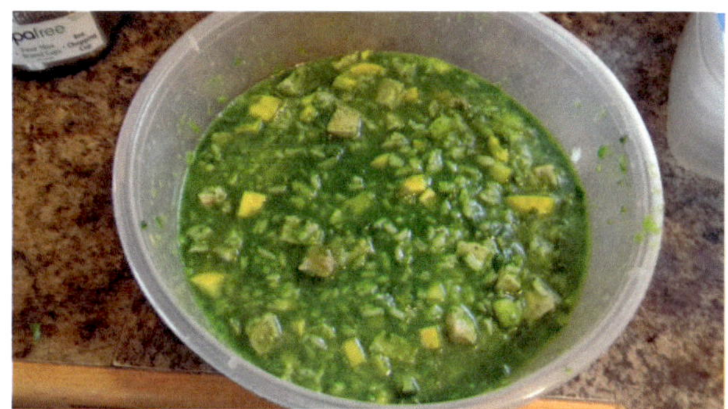

- 2 lbs of boneless pork cutlets
- 8 cups raw mustard greens
- 2 summer squash (yellow, but you can substitute zucchini if you want)
- 1 cup uncooked rice
- 2 Tbsp Flax seed oil
- 2000 mg calcium citrate
- water

Directions

Place the pork cutlets in a large pot and just cover with water. Bring to a boil then reduce heat and simmer for 15 minutes. Remove from heat and let cool a bit.

Microwave the summer squash on high for 3 minutes. Roll them over and microwave on high for another 3 minutes. Let cool enough to handle.

Place the mustard greens in a blender with ½ cup of water and finely chop or puree. Warning, when you puree mustard greens they give off a strong odor, this will dissipate, but don't stick your face right down near the blender top when you open it. This can make your eyes burn.

Remove the pork from the broth and dice up 3 cups of the meat. Put the broth in a large bowl.

Put 2½ cups of water in the large pot. Bring to a boil and add the rice. Reduce heat to a simmer, cover and cook for 5 minutes. This will leave the rice a little soupy, pour the rice into the bowl with your broth.

Remove the squash from the microwave, trim off the stem caps and flower nub and discard. Slice the squash in half lengthwise. Remove seeds with a spoon and discard, then dice the squash. Add diced squash to the large bowl.

Add the flax seed oil and calcium citrate to the bowl and mix well.

Add the pork and greens puree and stir in.

Seal and store in the fridge.

NOTES:

Whitefish, Zucchini, and Rice

A mild flavored stew

Ingredients

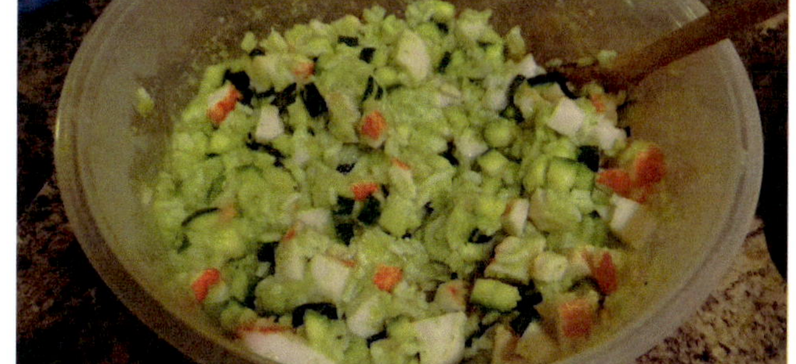

- 1 lb cooked white fish (I used faux crab)
- 3 zucchini
- 1 stalk of broccoli
- 1 cup uncooked rice
- 4 cups water

Directions

If your fish is not pre-cooked, cook it. Cut fish meat into chunks, you'll need 3 cups of cooked, chopped meat.

Put 2½ cups of water in a medium sauce pan and bring to a boil. Add 1 cup of raw rice. Return to boil, reduce heat to low, cover, and simmer for 15 minutes. Remove from heat and let sit a few minutes.

Place zucchini in the microwave and cook for 3 minutes on high. Roll them over and repeat. Remove and cut in half lengthwise. Scoop out seeds with a spoon and discard seeds. Dice the zucchini into ¼ inch cubes.

NOTE: When I did this recipe one of the 6 dogs was so totally averse to the diced zucchini that she would pick the diced pieces out and toss them on the floor. Fortunately the other dogs liked them and would clean up after her. But if you have a vegetable averse dog, mash the zucchini.

Chop the whole broccoli stalk, steam it in the microwave, and place it in a blender/food processor with ½ cup water. Chop on low. If the mix is too stiff to blend well, add more water. When you are done you will have 1 cup PLUS whatever amount of water you put in as puree. If you used ½ cup of water you should end up with 1½ cup of mush or puree to get the required 1 cup of broccoli.

Place the rice in a large bowl and mash. Add the zucchini and broccoli and mix through. Add a little water of it's too stiff. Add the fish and stir.

Place in an airtight container and store in the fridge.

NOTES:

The Template System

You may have noticed that many of these recipes use the same basic design template and plug different components into that template. There are four basic components:

Protein

Lean muscle meats such as pork, chicken, beef, fish or low-fat cheese.
3 cups total of either meat or meat and cheese mix.

Orange Vegetables

Sweet potato, any kind of squash, pumpkin, occasionally carrots (starchy)
3 cups when cooked and chopped or mashed.

Dark Green Vegetables

Spinach, Broccoli, Green pepper, Kale, Turnip greens, Mustard greens, etc.

You need 1 cup of finely chopped or pureed vegetable. Pureeing requires water to be added to facilitate blending (except for green peppers, they contain lots of water), so count that into the final product. Most greens will take 3 to 4 cups of raw vegetable. Steam it to soften, chop in a food processor or add enough water to allow it to puree. To get it right, if you added ½ cup of water, you need to end up with 1½ cups of puree (1 cup vegetable, ½ cup water)

Good Grains

Oats, rice, quinoa, barley, sorghum (avoid corn, wheat and soy)
You need to end up with three cups of cooked grain, then mash it

To avoid developing food allergies (and boredom) and to provide a better balanced diet, make each batch different by making selecting differing items from each of the four categories. Your dog(s) will show a preference toward certain items (mine are partial to sweet potato) and there is nothing wrong with catering to that preference most of the time, but do change it out occasionally to avoid problems.

Additives

To really spice things up you can add small amounts of other things to bring in additional nutrients and flavors. These include fruit like apple, orange, pears; other vegetables like tomato or carrot; other proteins like egg and yogurt; organ meats, especially chicken and beef heart, liver, and gizzards.

You might use a spoonful or two of any of these as a topping to add a little extra without compromising the overall formula.

Most of these recipes include calcium citrate and flax seed oil to keep things balanced. See Chapter 1 for details.

Chapter 8: Home-made Dog Treats

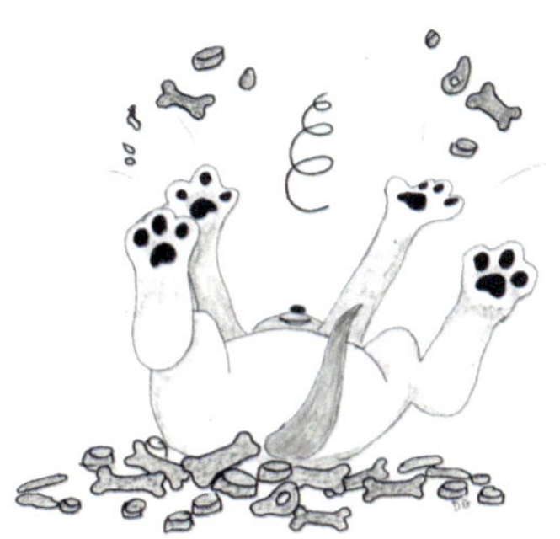

Regardless of how you choose to feed your dog his or her primary diet, home made dog treats are easy to make, fun to do, and hold just that much extra love for your companion. They are healthier than most commercially made treats too!

The recipes that follow have been selected because they are easy, healthy, and because our taste testers LOVED them. We know yours will too.

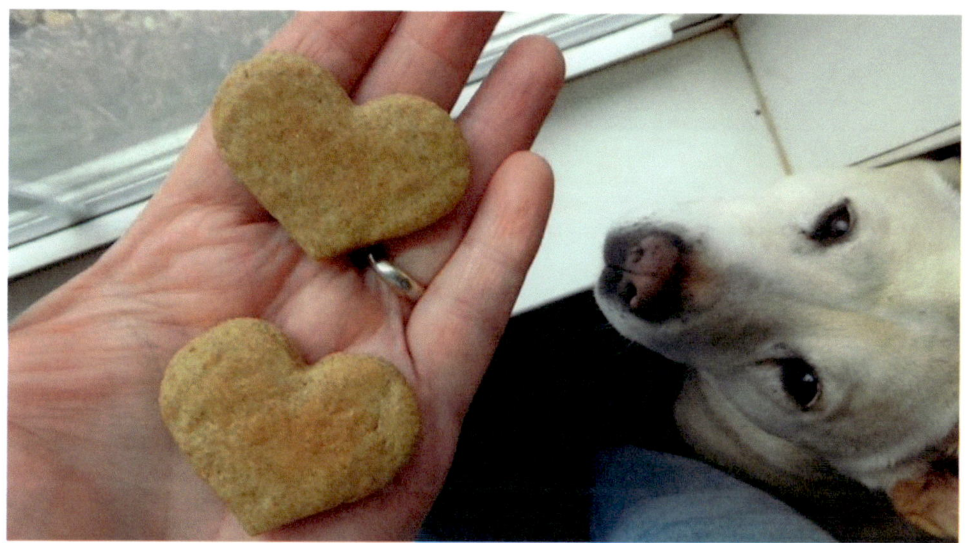

NOTES:

Buckwheat and Sweet Potato Dog Treats

You may have noticed that more and more people are turning up saying they have a gluten intolerance and are in need of gluten free foods. Oddly enough, DOGS are also becoming gluten intolerant. On this front, Marie has been experimenting with buckwheat.

Personally, I don't think it's the wheat that's the problem but the herbicides and insecticides (poisons) that are sprayed on the wheat (in America) that are the problem. I've read several accounts of gluten intolerant Americans who went to Europe on vacation and found they could eat all the European bread they wanted without any gastric upset. But that's not what this chapter is about.

If your dog has been diagnosed with gluten intolerance, many commercially available dog treats are off limits. Here's one you can make at home and your dog will enjoy. It uses buckwheat flour, but buckwheat is gluten free because it's not wheat. In fact it's not even a grain. I'd explain how that works, but that's not what his chapter is about either.

Best of all, these buckwheat dog treats can be super easy to make. You can make them more complicated, but you don't have to.

What You Need

First off, you're going to need some buckwheat flour. This can be had in the Natural or Organic sections of better grocery stores. If you can't find it, it is available from Amazon.com. We ordered a 5 pound box of Bob's Red Mill Organic Buckwheat from Amazon and got it at a favorable price. Because we are Prime members, shipping was free: that helps because ... 5 POUNDS! We like Bob's Red Mill products and have been pleased with this one too. What we got was 4, 22 ounce bags packaged in a box. It is interesting to note that a single 22 ounce bag was selling, at that time, for $9.86 and the box of four bags (same exact product) sold for $15.67. You do the math, but we thought this was a great value!

You can make these cookies with sweet potato, pumpkin, or squash and keep the high-fiber aspect. You can make your own by microwaving the vegetable until tender, scoop it out and puree it in a blender; adding just enough water to get the right consistency. Careful, though: not too much!

If you don't have time for that, you can use canned sweet potato, pumpkin, or squash. Just watch the labels and look for a low-sodium and no preservatives brand. Also, do NOT use pumpkin pie filling because this contains nutmeg and allspice, which are bad for dogs[9]. Nutmeg is known to cause hallucinations, seizures, and tremors in dogs. Allspice and cloves cause liver toxicity in cats. Granted, these occur when large amounts of spices are ingested; the traces used in baking *should* be safe. But since these are not for the discriminating palates of humans and dogs are more interested in the flavor of the prime ingredients, I'd play it safe and leave these out.

Let's Get Started

1. Preheat your oven to 350°
2. Line a cookie sheet with parchment paper
3. Add 1 Tbsp of raw honey to 8 ounces of pureed sweet potato (or pumpkin or squash) and mix through.
4. Mix 2 cups of buckwheat flour into the vegetable puree a little at a time. This will form a stiff dough, but because it's not sticky it's easy to work with. You will need to abandon the spoon and use your hands to mix in the last of the flour.
5. Roll the dough out on a floured surface. Roll it to just under 1/4" thickness for nice crunchy treats.
6. Use a cookie cutter to cut out shapes or cut the dough into rectangles with a pizza cutter.
7. Place cookies on the parchment-lined cookie sheet and bake at 350° for 25 minutes.
8. Remove and cool on a rack. Allow them to cool completely before handing out samples.

To store these treats, place them in an unsealed container like a pasteboard box (empty cereal box) or an old fashioned cookie jar. This will keep them crunchy. Sealing them into a plastic bag or sealed glass jar makes them get soft.

These can be safely stored at room temperature for a few days. If you will be using them slowly, bag some and freeze them, keeping out enough for no more than a week's worth of treats.

These treats have earned the paws up seal of approval from our dogs, Cochise, Blondie Bear, Josephine and Buddy Beagle. We gave some to our veterinarian, Dr. Sandra Manes DVM who says her dogs also love them. She was impressed enough with them to make a batch to take to a veterinarian thing she was going to that covered food intolerance and allergies in animals. We think that's a great endorsement!

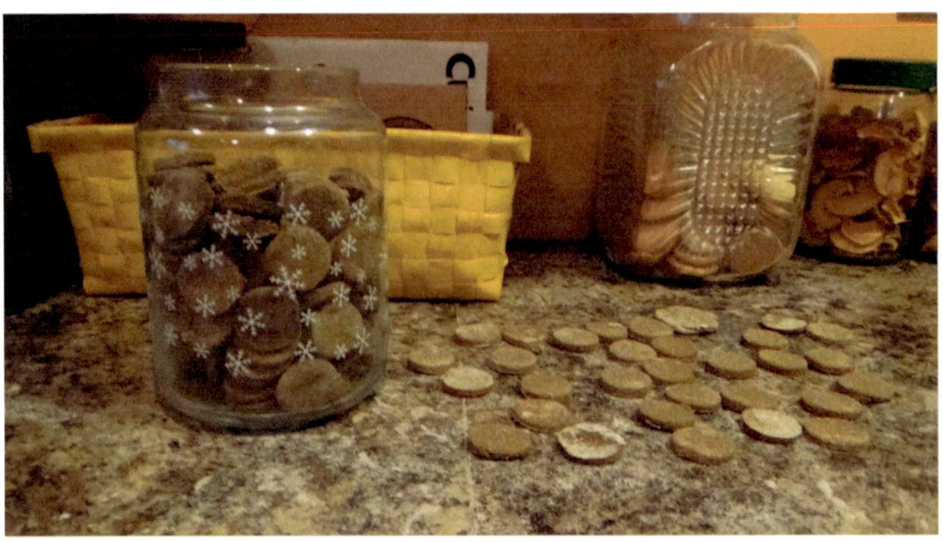

Peanut Butter Nummies

A large part of my rural life involves dogs. Not so much as working breeds – although mine do serve as mentors and tattletales – but more because my wife and I serve as a foster home for sick or wayward dogs. We work with the local animal shelter to help save some of their dogs from an untimely death.

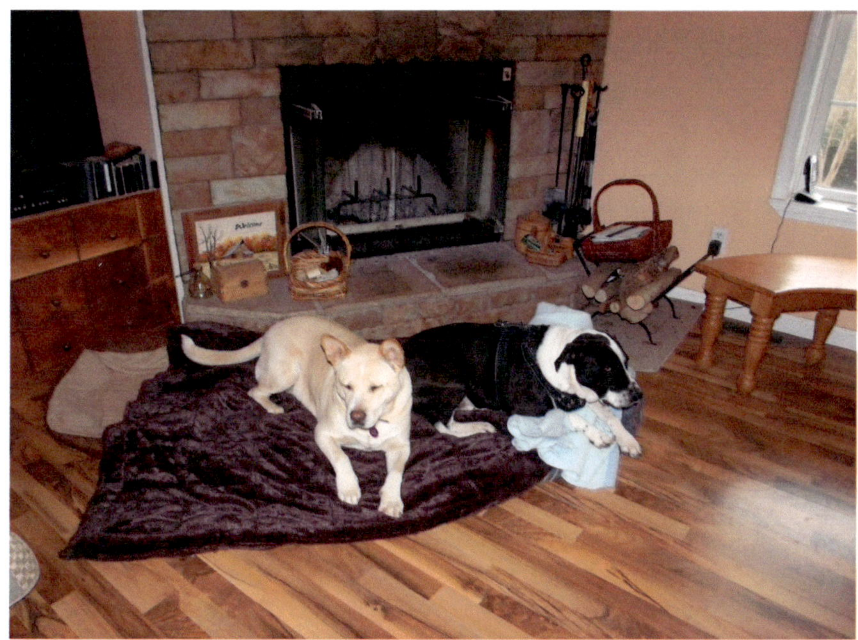

Our own dogs, Blondie and Cochise, were rescue dogs that we adopted. They are both excellent companions. While they may never herd sheep or guard chickens (mostly because we have neither), they do help us in mentoring the hooligan dogs that come into our program needing 'behavioral modification.'

Because they are such good members of our family, and helpful in our volunteer work, we spoil them just a bit. Part of that spoiling involves daily treats. Some are earned; some are just because we love them.

Recently there has been a flap about commercially made dog treats being tainted with all manner of unsavory things. Many dogs have been made very sick or died as a result. So I decided to strap on my apron and take a stab at making my own doggie treats.

Credit Where Credit is Due

I found this recipe floating around on the Internet. The poster said it originally came from Paula Dean's website. I've modified that to comply with what I have on hand to work with. Below is my version.

Prep Time: 15 min
Cook Time: 40 min

Difficulty: Easy-peasy

Ingredients:

- 3/4 cup milk
- 1 egg
- 1 cup smooth peanut butter
- 2 1/4 cups flour
- 1 tablespoon baking powder

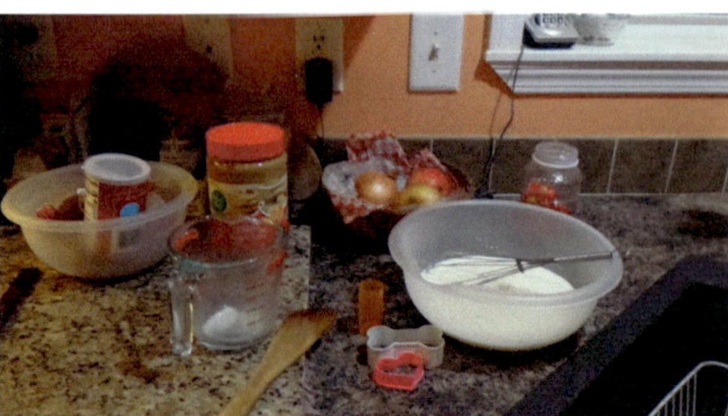

Directions:

Preheat oven to 325 F.

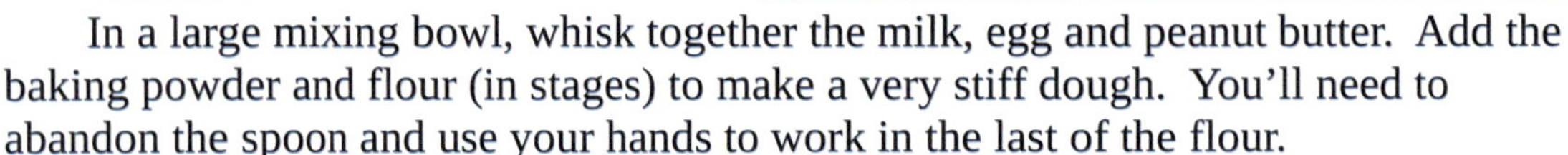

In a large mixing bowl, whisk together the milk, egg and peanut butter. Add the baking powder and flour (in stages) to make a very stiff dough. You'll need to abandon the spoon and use your hands to work in the last of the flour.

Flour a work surface and roll out dough to a 1/4-inch thickness. Thicker dough yields softer biscuits, for crunchy biscuits, stick to the 1/4-inch thickness. Cut into desired sizes (or use a cookie cutter) based on the size of your dog.

Bake on a parchment-lined baking tray for approximately 20 minutes (a little longer for harder biscuits). Turn biscuits over and bake for an additional 15 minutes. Move from cooking sheet to a cooling rack and allow them to cool completely before storing in an airtight container.

Observations

I used a biscuit cutter, which yielded about 2 dozen biscuits that are 2 1/4 inches in diameter: a suitable size for our 80-pound bulldogs. OK, they're closer to 90 pounds: too many cookies, not enough running in the yard. Spring is coming (one of these days), and we'll rectify that second part.

I have since switched to using a smaller cookie cutter. This yields a treat that is just under 1 inch in diameter and is far more suitable for use as a training treat and as incentive for crating.

Do they like them? Do they ever!

In fact after a few days of these cookies, I offered Cochise a commercial dog cookie. He eyed it suspiciously, sniffed at it, gingerly took it between two teeth, dropped it to the floor, looked at it, then at me, "You don't expect me to eat THAT do you?"

Did I mention they're a little spoiled?

Easy Peasy Cheesy Dog Cookies

Dogs love cheese, so even the most discriminating dog ought to love these cheesy dog treats. Because they're homemade and you will choose the ingredients, you know they contain nothing insidious — something you can't be sure of with commercial treats. They're easy to make, too! Because they're made with real cheese they add protein to your dogs diet, but they ARE treats: so dispense responsibly.

Ingredients

- 1/2 cup shredded cheddar cheese
- 1/2 cup shredded Parmesan cheese
- 3 tablespoons flax seed oil
- 1 1/2 cup whole wheat flour
- 1/2 cup + 1 Tbsp low fat milk

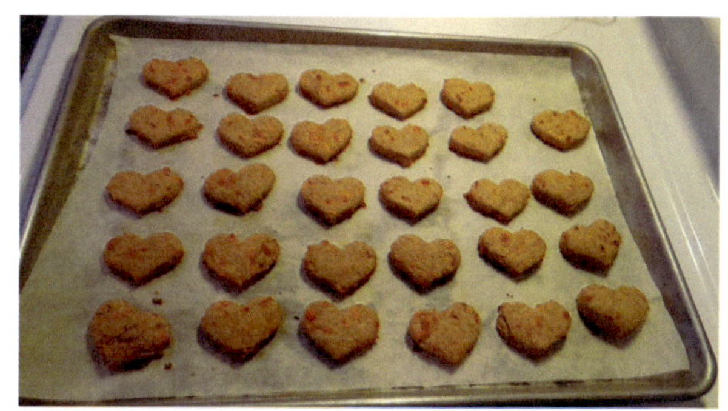

Preparing Cheesy Dog Treats

Preheat oven to 350 degrees F. Line a baking sheet with parchment paper.

In a large bowl, mix cheeses with oil. Stir in flour gradually until blended. Mix in milk and knead until dough comes together.

Roll dough on a lightly floured surface to 1/4 inch thickness,

Cut out treats using a cookie cutter or juice glass (or just cut the dough unto squares with a pizza cutter, if you're lazy).

Gather the scraps into a clump and repeat 3, 4, and 5 until all dough is used.

Bake for 30 minutes, or until treats are golden brown.

Makes 16, 2 inch diameter treats (plus that little oddball bit). Using a smaller cutter makes more treats. The 2″ are perfect for our big bullies, smaller are better for the Beagles.

These cute 2″ x 1.5″ hearts turned out to be a great compromise. And I got 30 of them per batch.

Allow your cheesy dog treats to cool thoroughly before serving to your furry friend(s). After they've completely cooled, store in a zip-lock bag or a jar. They'll be okay at room temperature for a day or two, but because there are no preservatives, keep the bag in the fridge after that (if there any left) to prevent mold. If you're real stingy, freeze them for long-term storage.

Because the dough is quite stiff, if you want to make more at one time, make several batches instead of doubling the ingredients and making a larger batch.

NOTES:

Chapter 9: Special Needs Diets

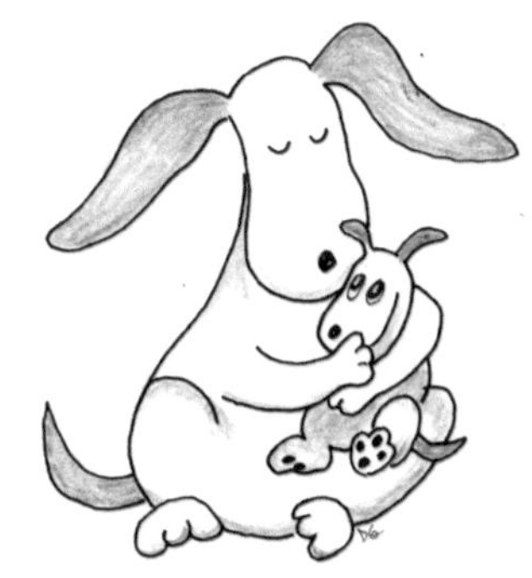

Dogs, as do people, sometimes suffer physical problems that require special diets: diabetes, allergies, cancer, weak heart, pancreatitis, kidney failure, and obesity are among the most common. This section will offer recipes for dog food that helps you deal with these physical problems. Because these are special needs diets, I have not tested them on my own dogs, but they have been reviewed and approved by Dr. Sandra Manes DVM. Any commentary she had is also included. I highly recommend that you work closely with your veterinarian as you decide on diet so testing can be done to see what effect you're having on body chemistry.

Diabetes

Anyone who is diabetic, be they canine or human, will do better with a diet of appealing food so their daily intake is consistent and predictable. The diet fed to diabetic dogs should remain nutritionally balanced. In this section we pay special attention to those elements that produce sugars (aka blood glucose or a glycemic response) in your dog's body.

For reasons discussed in the GRAINS section of this book, we want to avoid corn, wheat, and soy in diabetic recipes. Many I've seen use rice instead but, as it turns out, even brown rice is a poor choice for the diabetic dog diet.

Dr. Sandra Manes DVM cites a study done on dietary carbohydrate response in diabetic and non-diabetic dogs. In commercial dog food, the processing method has minimal influence on the post-feeding glycemic levels. The major glycemic influence is the <u>source</u> of the dietary carbs.

In non-diabetic dogs, a sorghum based diet ("based" refers to the source of the carbohydrates, not as being the primary component of the food) resulted in the lowest post-feeding *glucose* response. A barley based diet produced the lowest post-feeding *insulin* response. And a rice based diet resulted in significantly higher post-feeding glucose and insulin responses.

Especially for diabetic dogs being treated with fixed, daily doses of insulin (not using frequent blood tests and a sliding insulin scale) it is necessary to provide a consistent level of dietary carbohydrate each day. Foods providing carbohydrates through rice should be avoided in diabetic dogs, while sorghum and barley are more suitable carbohydrate sources.

I'm sure you've seen barley in the stores: it's used frequently in soups. Sorghum is also a "grass" (technically it is not a grain, although package labels often describe it as such) the seed or kernel of which can be bought whole kernel, ground into meal or flour, or made into flakes and sold as breakfast cereal. You may have to look in the gluten-free section of your grocery store to find it.

Because canine diabetes often develops with a form of pancreatitis that is not severe enough to present definite or readily observable symptoms, some veterinarians will put a dog on a low fat diet to forestall full blown (clinical) pancreatitis. However, clinical studies show random results for such dietary changes: it helps some dogs, in others it leads to undesirable weight loss without affecting the lipid counts as hoped. Keep your veterinarian in the loop and monitoring these elements of your dog's blood.

With all that in mind, let's look at some recipes.

Ground Meat Stew

This recipe makes about 2 gallons of food. If you do not have large pans or a stock pot cut down the amounts to suit your pans.

You should vary both the meat and vegetables used in each batch you make depending on what is inexpensive. This provides a better balanced diet over the long term and avoid food allergies. For diabetics do not use corn, carrots, peas, or potato as the vegetable - nothing with carbohydrates. Dark green or orange vegetables are highest in vitamins.

Ingredients

- 6 pounds lean ground beef, chicken, or other lean meat
- 6,000 mg of Calcium Citrate or 3 Tbsp bone meal
- 5 cups uncooked pearl barley
- 5 cups uncooked sorghum
- 2 cups minced celery, green beans, chopped spinach (or other dark green vegetable)
- 28 cups water. (Sorghum takes 3 cups of water per cup of uncooked grain. The barley takes slightly more than 2 cups per, so use 28 cups.)

Directions

1. Open the calcium capsules and mix it through the raw ground meat.
2. Put ingredients in large Dutch oven or stock pot and bring to a boil.
3. Lower heat to a simmer, cover and cook until all the water is absorbed.
4. Stir to mix well. Divide for storage and refrigerate or freeze.

Turkey and Oats

- 12 cups water
- 6 cups raw rolled oats
- 3 pounds (6 cups) raw ground or chopped turkey
- 6 cups raw dark green, orange (not carrots) and/or red vegetables
- 1½ tablespoons bone meal (or 3,000 mg calcium citrate)
- 10,000 IU vitamin A
- 400 IU vitamin E

Directions

Bring the water to a boil.

Mix the calcium through your meat.

Add turkey and oats to the boiling water and reduce heat to a simmer and cover. Cook until liquid is absorbed, stirring frequently.

While the oats and meat cook, steam or microwave your veggies until soft, then puree or mash thoroughly.

Add vitamins to vegetable mash and stir through.

When the oat mixture is done remove from heat and mix vegetable mash in, stir thoroughly.

Divide for storage and refrigerate.

Chicken and Broccoli

A small-batch recipe great for small dogs or if you don't have space to store gallons of dog food.

Ingredients

- 3 skinless whole chicken breasts (approx 1 lb of meat)
- 8 cups water
- 1 lg head of broccoli
- 3 cups barley (dry)
- 1000 mg calcium citrate or ½ Tbsp of bone meal

Directions

Boil the chicken in water until cooked through.

Remove the cooked chicken (save the broth), cool the chicken and cut into small pieces.

Cook the barley in 7 cups of the saved broth for 20 to 25 minutes. Mash the barley.

Steam or microwave the broccoli and mash well or puree.

Combine all ingredients (including the calcium) and mix well. If it looks dry, add more of the saved broth.

Diabetic Dog Treats

Recipe by Barb Maxwell as posted on AllRecipes.com

Ingredients

- ½ cup whole wheat flour
- 2 eggs
- 1½ pounds beef liver cut into pieces

Directions

Preheat oven to 350° F.

Line a 10" x 15" jelly roll pan with parchment paper

Place liver into a food processor and pulse until finely chopped.

Add flour and eggs, process until smoooth.

Note: If there is not enough room to process the whole batch, remove ½ the liver, add 1 egg and ¼ cup flour and process. Move this to a bowl and repeat with the rest of the ingredients. Mix well in the bowl.

Spread this mixture evenly in the prepared pan.

Bake for 15 minutes or until the center is firm.

Cool, then turn out onto a cutting board and cut into squares sized to suit your dog with a pizza cutter. This treat has the consistency of a sponge.

Store in an airtight container in the fridge.

Obesity

The key to feeding an obese dog is to eliminate fat content and limit starches that turn to sugar and are stored as fat, without depriving the dog of other needed dietary elements.

Of course increasing the dogs physical activity will go a long way toward trimming him down too. This may be difficult at first, but as the weight starts to come off most dogs will become more active.

Recipes should focus on lean meats, low starch grains, and avoid cheese or peanut butter. Also avoid white potatoes, peas, green beans, and corn which are starchy vegetables.

See the Grains section of Chapter 2 for details of which grains to use.

You can use any of the template recipes listed in this book, just use these recommendations in choosing the specific components.

Kidney Disease

It is absolutely vital that a dog with kidney disease be fed a diet that will not put further stress on their kidneys. The main goal of a homemade canine kidney diet is to feed your dog as little phosphorus as possible. The exact amount depends on the stage of your dog's kidney disease, so consult your vet for more details, but 10 milligram per pound of body weight is the limit for dogs with advanced renal failure. In the broadest sense, this means that the diet must consist of foods with lower levels of: sugar, fat, protein, potassium as well as phosphorous. On the other hand, the following foods should be included in your dog's homemade diet:

- Boiled rice
- Chicken and duck are good for protein/phosphorus balance in kidney diseased dogs
- Chicken liver
- Research shows, and vets recommend, a dog kidney disease diet should have up to 50% in carbs. They're a good source of calories for dogs with CKD because most foods will be low in phosphorous. These foods will include vegetables (like corn, peas, and green beans) and fruits, as well as appropriate grains.
- Cornflour is a type of flour that's milled from dried whole corn kernels. It contains the hull, germ, and endosperm of the corn and is considered a whole grain flour.
- Peanut butter contains vitamins H and E. Vitamin H improves the sheen in a dog's coat, strengthens the nails and is good for the skin. Vitamin E is an immune system enhancer. These factors make it a good treat for dogs with

kidney disease since the dog's coat will become less healthy and the dog will have a decreased ability to fight off infection.

- When feeding a homemade diet, foods like liver, tuna packed in oil, and salmon will supply vitamin D3.
- Include omega-3s. Studies have shown that supplementation with omega-3 fatty acids can help the function of kidneys, and assist with dog kidney disease in general. This includes feeding foods higher in omega-3 fatty acids, like fish, or using flax seed oil and fish oil as supplements in the food.

Heart Disease

Taurine is an amino acid important for heart health. Taurine deficiency has been known for many years to lead to dilated cardiomyopathy, or DCM, a heart muscle disorder that can lead to congestive heart failure and death. Recently "boutique" pet foods containing peas, lentils, other legume seeds, or potatoes as main ingredients, are what's being linked to DCM, which leads to reduced heart pumping function and increased heart size. The alterations in heart function and structure can result in severe consequences.

In a dog suffering from DCM, boosting taurine intake can help. Organ meats like heart and kidney are good sources of taurine. Adding an increased percentage of these to your recipes can help maintain your dog's heart.

In July of 2018, the FDA announced it had begun investigating reports of DCM in dogs eating certain diets. Many of the implicated diets were labeled as 'grain-free', and contained peas, lentils, other legume seeds, and/or potatoes (as primary ingredients)[21].

Recently, the focus has shifted to an association between grain-free diets and the development of DCM in our canine patients. More specifically, the implicated diets are collectively referred to as 'BEG diets' from Boutique companies, contain Exotic ingredients, and many are labeled as Grain-free. Veterinary cardiologists across the country have been diagnosing increased rates of DCM in dogs eating these diets, with many dogs showing improvement when the diet is changed. This recent association has resulted in many concerned owners and veterinarians alike.

An update on the investigation was released in June 2019. This update detailed 574 reported cases of DCM between January 2014 and April 2019 (560 dogs and 14 cats). The reported cases included a wide range of breeds, many without a genetic predisposition to developing DCM. Some of the cases showed evidence of low blood taurine levels, while others had normal or high blood taurine levels. Of the reported cases, more than 90% of the diets were labeled as 'grain-free', and 93% of the diets contained peas and/or lentils as a main ingredient. A much smaller proportion of diets contained potatoes. Many of the pets were fed exclusively dry food (86%), with smaller numbers eating wet/dry combinations, raw diets, or homecooked diets. The animal protein sources in the diets varied greatly. A list of the most frequently named dog food brands in the reported cases can be observed in Figure 1 (next page).

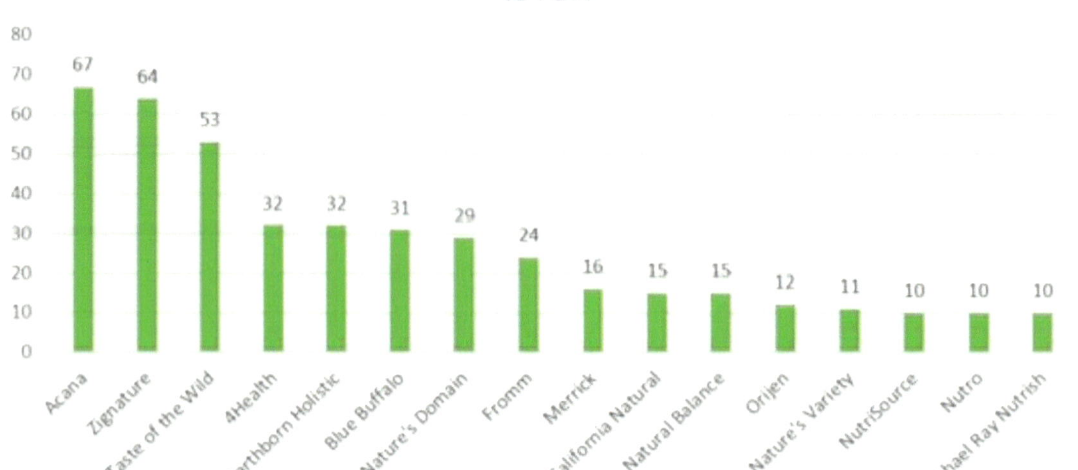

Congestive Heart Failure (CHF) is a little different in that the main enemy is sodium, which causes fluid retention in and around the heart. Doing everything you can to reduce sodium is helpful at this stage.

Because dogs with heart disease tend to be more sedentary, they gain weight early on. Avoiding starchy vegetables and fatty meats helps with this. Later, the dog loses his or her appetite and may not take in enough nourishment to maintain health. This is where a home cooked diet really shines, because most dogs much prefer it to a commercial diet.

Cancer

When your dog is suffering from cancer, experts suggest to avoid carbohydrates and use moderate protein levels. Because bacteria is a concern, be sure to cook recipes to reduce bacteria.

One option is to mix:

- 1 cup cooked brown rice
- 2 soft-scrambled eggs (note: be sure the whites are cooked through, yolks can be soft)
- 1 teaspoon flax seed oil
- 1 cup steamed vegetables, pureed in a blender or food processor (healthy vegetables include zucchini, squash, cauliflower, broccoli, peas and spinach)
- 1/2 cup cottage cheese

- 1/2 cup protein, such as diced beef, chicken or turkey

This will feed a small dog for a day. For a medium sized dog, double it. Triple the recipe for a large dog.

Pancreatitis

This is not something you should take on by yourself. Your veterinarian or a nutritionist recommended by your vet should be closely involved in designing meals for your dog.

But generally speaking, a dog with pancreatitis needs to be on a low-fat diet with plenty of carbohydrates. The dog should be fed several times a day to maintain nutrient and electrolyte balances in the bloodstream. Many veterinarians recommend three daily feedings. If the vomiting is severe and medication is being used to control nausea and vomiting, wait a day before offering a small meal. Encourage water intake by tempting the dog with meat-flavored water or by purchasing a pet drinking fountain.

Common ingredients include, turkey, chicken, barley, brown rice, flax seed, and potatoes. So meals are not out of your scope, but it's important to follow the nutritionist's advice. Homemade foods must have the proper ratios of meat and high-quality carbohydrates, as well as amino acid, vitamin and mineral supplements. But these ratios vary with you dog's progress through the disease.

Thank You

I want to thank you for purchasing this book. All proceeds from sales of this book go to Piney Mountain Foster Care, Inc. a 501(c)(3) public charity.

Piney Mountain Foster Care is a small, all volunteer, non-profit kennel facility located on 4 acres of mountainside property in Edwina Tennessee. We got our start in 2012 by caring for dogs going through heart worm treatment. We still do this and other medical care. We also work with dogs with behavioral issues. But we are delighted to work with well-adjusted, healthy dogs who just need a break in life.

Our primary mission is to help rescue dogs from kill shelters. Many need health care. Most need training. That's where we come in. We offer medical rehabilitation and behavioral modification in a tranquil setting.

When adoptable, we work with and through canine rescues locally and around the nation to find these dogs quality homes. See the Canine Rescue Partners page of our web site for details on them.

The secondary mission is to raise awareness and promote prevention of animal cruelty and to curb rampant companion animal over-population by promoting low cost spay-neuter programs.

For more information on Piney Mountain Foster Care, go to:

https://PineyMountainFoster.org

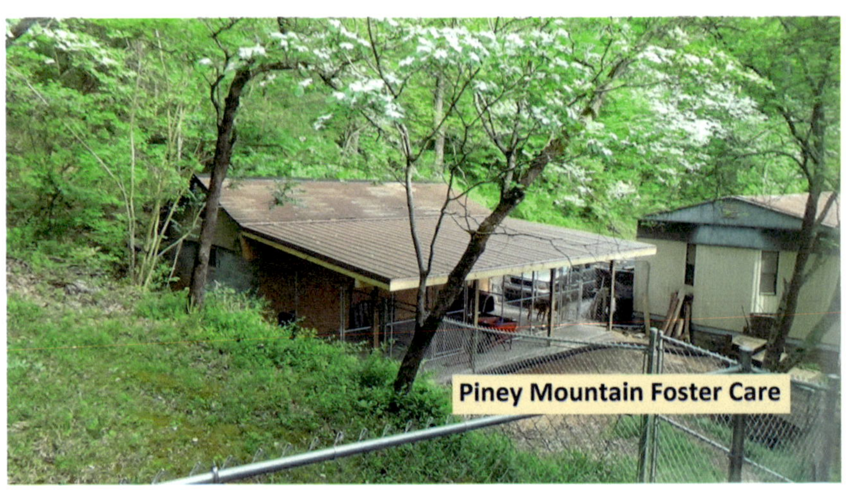

Resources:

1. ASPCA: https://www.aspca.org/
2. Pet Food Safety Center – Humane Society: http://www.humanesociety.org/animals/resources/facts/pet_food_safety.html
3. American Academy of Veterinary Nutrition: http://www.aavn.org/nutrition-resources/
4. Dr. Sandra Manes DVM, Cedarwood Veterinary Hospital, Newport TN.
5. USDA Food and Nutrition Information Center https://www.nal.usda.gov/fnic
6. SELF Nutrition Data http://nutritiondata.self.com
7. Dog Food Adviser http://dogfoodadviser.com
8. Dog Food Insider https://www.dogfoodinsider.com
9. Pets with Diabetes: http://www.petdiabetes.com
10. Whole Dog Journal
11. *Home Cooking For Your Dog* (Abrams) by Christine M. Filardi
12. *Dr. Pitcairn's Complete Guide to Natural Health for Dogs & Cats* (Rodale Press) by Dr. Richard H. Pitcairn DVM
13. Vet Info web site http://www.VetInfo.com
14. Today's Veterinarian Practice: https://todaysveterinarypractice.com
15. Animal Wellness Magazine
16. "Quinoa: An ancient crop to contribute to world food security" (PDF). Food and Agriculture Organization. July 2011. Retrieved 22 May 2018.
17. A Novices Guide to Raw Feeding for Dogs: https://keepthetailwagging.com/noviceguide
18. Pros and Cons of the BARF Diet for Dogs: https://topdogtips.com/barf-diet-for-dogs/
19. Dog and Cat Food Recipes: http://dish.allrecipes.com/homemade-pet-food/
20. Allrecipes.com recipes reprinted with permission from Meredith Publications
21. https://www.medvetforpets.com/beg-diets-and-dcm-in-dogs-recommendations-regarding-diagnosis-and-management/
22. https://www.veterinarypracticenews.com/research-updates-on-diet-associated-dilated-cardiomyopathy-2/
23. https://www.dvm360.com/view/journal-scan-dcm-and-boutique-dog-foods-can-taurine-supplementation-help

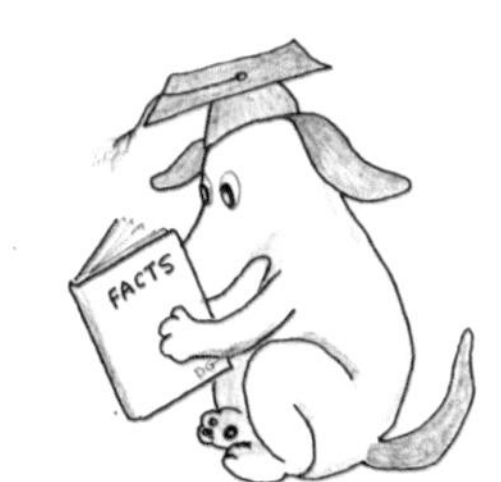

NOTES:

Made in the USA
Columbia, SC
18 March 2025

55357480R00060